"This book is an essential read for anyone considering, starting, or developing their career as a psychological practitioner. What sets this book apart is its inclusive approach. It is written by experienced practitioners who have ensured that they involved the very workforce they are representing which conveys a sense of authenticity from the outset. This book not only considers the journey of becoming a psychological practitioner, but it gives the reader a real sense of what it is like to work as psychological practitioner."

Paul Thompson, *Teesside University, UK*

Building a Career as a Psychological Practitioner

This useful and accessible guide introduces the reader to the psychological practitioner roles and offers practical advice for those looking to pursue a career in the wider psychological professions.

Demonstrating that psychology is not a 'one-size-fits-all' profession, Ward and Drysdale guide readers through the options and pathways for a successful career as a psychological practitioner, including as a psychological wellbeing practitioner (PWP), mental health wellbeing practitioner, children's wellbeing practitioner (CWP), and education mental health practitioner (EMHP). This book covers the entire process from moving into the profession and being a trainee to mastering the job market and making the most of your career and next steps. Bringing together these four important roles, this book offers a comprehensive overview while also allowing you to dip in and out of the chapters to access needed information quickly and easily.

Supported by an acronym decoder and real-life, diverse case studies, this is an indispensable resource for anyone looking to understand the potential of psychologically informed careers and move into a psychological practitioner role.

Elspeth Ward is currently a supervision lead across NHS Talking Therapies Mersey Care, a registered PWP and co-Chair of the Psychological Professions Network North West (PPN NW) Psychological Practitioner Community of Practice.

Kirsty Drysdale is a specialist lecturer on the CWP and EMHP programmes at the Psychological Therapies Training Centre in Manchester, a clinically practicing CWP, and a co-Chair of the PPN NW Psychological Practitioner Community of Practice.

BPS Pathways in Psychology Series
British Psychological Society

Routledge, in partnership with the British Psychological Society (BPS), is pleased to present *BPS Pathways in Psychology*, a new generation of informative books designed to support individuals looking to begin careers in or using psychology. Divided into two streams, the series offers titles both for those looking to follow a more traditional career route, or those who wish to understand how their psychology degree can inform their career outside a chartered role.

Making it clear that there is not a 'one size fits all' approach to a career in or using psychology, each book is supported by case studies that highlight diversity of voice and progression routes, anecdotal guidance on avoiding pitfalls, and further reading and resources.

These early career "bookshelf essential" texts provide accessible, evidence-based, practice-oriented guides for students and professionals.

Building a Career as a Psychological Practitioner
Elspeth Ward and Kirsty Drysdale

For more information about this series, please visit: https://www.routledge.com/our-products/book-series/BPSPIP

Building a Career as a Psychological Practitioner

Elspeth Ward and
Kirsty Drysdale

Routledge
Taylor & Francis Group

LONDON AND NEW YORK

Cover image credit: Nigel Turner

First published 2026
by Routledge
4 Park Square, Milton Park, Abingdon, Oxon OX14 4RN

and by Routledge
605 Third Avenue, New York, NY 10158

Routledge is an imprint of the Taylor & Francis Group, an informa business

For Product Safety Concerns and Information please contact
our EU representative GPSR@taylorandfrancis.com. Taylor &
Francis Verlag GmbH, Kaufingerstraße 24, 80331 München,
Germany.

Trademark notice: Product or corporate names may be trademarks
or registered trademarks, and are used only for identification and
explanation without intent to infringe.

British Library Cataloguing-in-Publication Data
A catalogue record for this book is available from
the British Library

ISBN: 9781032892689 (hbk)
ISBN: 9781032892672 (pbk)
ISBN: 9781003542049 (ebk)

DOI: 10.4324/9781003542049

Typeset in Optima
by codeMantra

Contents

Acknowledgements

Elspeth and Kirsty would like to thank all those who have inspired, taught, and encouraged them as they have progressed through their careers. These individuals know who, and how appreciated, they are.

The authors would also like to recognise and thank all trainee and qualified psychological practitioners across the roles, plus clinical supervisors, educators, line managers, and a wide range of other professionals who have contributed directly to this book:

Adam Hope – Qualified MHWP

Ally Boyne – Specialist Lecturer on EMHP and CWP programmes, and CBT Therapist

Amelia Bellmon – Qualified CWP, Associate Lecturer on CWP and EMHP programmes, Clinical Supervisor, and CBT Therapist

Amy Newton – Qualified CWP

Anna Dagnall – Specialist Lecturer on CWP, EMHP, and HI CBT programmes, Clinical Supervisor, and CBT Therapist

Anne Masterson – Qualified CWP

Bryony Beetham – Lecturer, Team Lead, and Qualified PWP

Charlotte Temple – Specialist Lecturer on CWP, EMHP, SWP, Supervisor, and HI CBT programmes, Clinical Supervisor, and CBT Therapist

Danielle Robinson – Qualified EMHP

Elle Crane – Qualified CWP, CBT Therapist, and Clinical Supervisor

Ellie McKelvey – Trainee CWP

Emma Ellis – Qualified EMHP

Eve Bampton-Wilton – Qualified PWP, Senior Lecturer, and Clinical Programme Manager in the PPN South West

Faye Whitehill – Qualified CWP

Gareth Edwards – Specialist Lecturer on CWP and EMHP programmes and CBT Therapist

Georgia Jameson – Trainee MHWP and Qualified APP

Georgina Shires – Specialist Lecturer on CWP, EMHP, Supervisor, and SWP programmes, Clinical Supervisor, and CBT Therapist

Grace Wiles – Trainee EMHP

Jasmine Pugh – Trainee EMHP

Jordan Howarth – Qualified PWP, HIT, and Supervision Lead

Julie Browne – Qualified EMHP, Associate Lecturer on CWP and EMHP programmes, and Clinical Supervisor

Karen Rea – PWP Programme Leader

Katie Jamieson – Qualified CWP and trainee SWP

Kelly DeSantis – LTC-trained PWP

Kirsten Brown – Qualified MHWP

Laura Spence – Qualified CWP

Lauren White – Qualified CWP

Lennie Jervis – Qualified CWP

Lettie Smyth – Qualified CWP

Lisa Buffel – Qualified CWP

Louise Britton – Qualified EMHP

Louise Rawley – Qualified EMHP

Madeleine Shimwell – Qualified PWP

Marianne Tay – MHWP Course Lead and CBT Therapist

Marin Cash – Qualified PWP

Matthew Beaton – Principal Mental Health Practitioner and Honorary Lecturer

Matthew Draper – Trainee CWP

Melissa Street – Consultant Psychological Therapist and former Programme Lead on CWP programme

Nick Jackson – Senior PWP

Nikki Nolan – Trainee EMHP

Paul Thompson – Senior Lecturer in Mental Health, and Director of the Psychological Professionals' Development Hub and qualified PWP,

Paula Mohin – Trainee CWP

Phillip Irlam – Qualified MHWP

Rebecca Somerville-Clegg – Qualified CWP

Rob Leigh – NHS TT Supervision Lead, qualified PWP, HI CBT Therapist, and EMDR Consultant

Robyn Ward – Qualified CWP, Clinical Supervisor, and Trainee HI CBT Therapist

Safa Asif – Qualified CWP

Sam Torney – NHS TT Team Lead, qualified PWP, and Chair BABCP Low-Intensity SIG

Samantha Taylor – Qualified CWP and trainee SWP

Sandi McGuire – Qualified CWP

Sara Yunus – MHST Service Lead, Specialist Lecturer on CWP programme, Clinical Supervisor, and CBT Therapist

Sarah Barker – PWP Clinical Lead and LTC-trained PWP

Sheldon Rodrigues – Senior PWP

Sian Clements – Senior PWP

Sophie Maylor – Qualified CWP

Stacy Smith – Qualified PWP and Team Lead

Susan Moore – Qualified CWP

Vongai Tepa – Qualified PWP

Acronym Decoder

The National Health Service (NHS) and psychological professions are renowned for being loaded with acronyms. This acronym decoder should help you understand the acronyms we have used and can be referred to as you read on

ADHD	Attention-Deficit Hyperactivity Disorder
AP	Assistant Psychologist
APP	Associate Psychological Practitioner
BA	Behavioural Activation
BABCP	British Association of Behavioural and Cognitive Psychotherapies
BBA	Brief Behavioural Activation
BPS	British Psychological Society
CAMHS	Child and Adolescent Mental Health Services
CBT	Cognitive Behavioural Therapy
cCBT	Computerised Cognitive Behavioural Therapy
CCMS	Clinical Case Management Supervision
CMS	Case Management Supervision
CLM	Caseload Management
CPD	Continuing Professional Development
CR	Cognitive Restructuring
CS	Clinical Skills
CSS	Clinical Skills Supervision
CWP	Children and Young People's Wellbeing Practitioner

CYP	Children and Young People (if in the context of a group) *or* Child or Young Person (if referring to an individual)
CYP IAPT	Children and Young People's Improving Access to Psychological Therapies
CYP PT	Children and Young People's Psychological Trainings
CYPMHS	Children and Young People's Mental Health Services
CYWP	North West–specific acronym for Children and Young People's Wellbeing Practitioner
D&A	Drug and Alcohol services
DMHL	Designated Mental Health Lead
EBSA	Emotionally Based School Avoidance
EDI	Equality, Diversity, and Inclusion
EHCP	Education Health and Care Plan
EIPT	Early Intervention in Psychosis Team
EIT	Early Intervention Team
EMDR	Eye Movement Desensitisation and Reprocessing
EMHP	Education Mental Health Practitioner
ERP	Exposure and Response Prevention
ETAP	Education Training Activity Plan
GAD	Generalised Anxiety Disorder
GCert	Graduate Certificate
GDip	Graduate Diploma
GE	Graded Exposure
GP	General Practitioner
HEE	Health Education England
HEI	Higher Education Institution
HRT	Habit Reversal Therapy
IAG	Information, Advice, and Guidance
IAPT	Improving Access to Psychological Therapies
ICB	Integrated Care Board
ICS	Integrated Care System
KPIs	Key Performance Indicators
KSBs	Knowledge, Skills, and Behaviours
LEAP	Lived Experience Advisory Panel
LGBTQ+	Lesbian, Gay, Bisexual, Transgender, Queer/Questioning plus (plus indicating wider

	sexualities/identities not covered by those listed)
LMS	Line Management Supervision
LTCs	Long-Term Conditions
LTP	Long-Term Plan
LTWP	Long-Term Workforce Plan
MDS	Minimum Data Set
MDT	Multidisciplinary Team
METIP	Multi-Professional Education and Training Investment Plan
METP	Multi-Professional Education and Training Plan
MHWP	Mental Health Wellbeing Practitioner
NAT	Negative Automatic Thought
NHS	National Health Service
NHS AfC	NHS Agenda for Change (pay scales)
NHSE	NHS England
NHSTT	NHS Talking Therapies
NHSTTad	NHS Talking Therapies for Anxiety and Depression
OCD	Obsessive Compulsive Disorder
OSCE	Observed Structured Clinical Examination
PBL	Problem Based Learning
PGCert	Postgraduate Certificate
PGDip	Postgraduate Diploma
PP	Psychological Practitioner
PROMs	Patient-Reported Outcome Measure/Measurement
PSA	Professional Standards Authority
PSAD	Practice Skills Assessment Document
PTSD	Post-Traumatic Stress Disorder
PWP	Psychological Wellbeing Practitioner
QI	Quality Improvement
RIA	Recent Incident Analysis
ROMs	Routine Outcome Measures/Measurement
SMHL	Senior Mental Health Lead
SPWP	Senior Psychological Wellbeing Practitioner
SWP	Senior Wellbeing Practitioner
TAPP	Trainee Associate Psychological Practitioner
TIC	Trauma Informed Care

VCSE	Voluntary, Community, and Social Enterprise services
WAP	Widening Access and Participation
WM	Worry Management
WSA	Whole School Approach
YIAC Service	Youth Information Advice and Counselling Service
YIPP	Youth Intensive Psychological Practitioner
YP	Young People (if in the context of a group) *or* Young Person (if referring to an individual)

Chapter 1

Introduction and How to Use This Book

Introduction

The psychological practitioner (PP) roles, which include the role of Psychological Wellbeing Practitioner (PWP), Mental Health Wellbeing Practitioner (MHWP), Children's Wellbeing Practitioner (CWP), and Education Mental Health Practitioner (EMHP), are linked through their offer of low-intensity, cognitive behavioural therapy (CBT) informed support and intervention. The PWP and MHWP roles work with adults, whilst the CWP and EMHP roles work with children, young people (YP), and families.

Each of these roles provides new and exciting opportunities to increase access to psychologically informed careers, as well as broadening psychologically informed treatment options for clients, children, YP, and families. Psychology is not a 'one-size-fits-all' profession. People are individual, and our careers, and the treatment options these provide, need to reflect the populations we serve. In this book, your authors, Elspeth and Kirsty, will guide you through the roles and options for a rewarding and interesting career as a PP.

But first, why have we written this book? The PP roles are often less well known outside of the immediate profession. If there is limited information out there about the roles, how can we encourage people to train and work in them? For potential trainees, how do you know which career path is right for you without having access to information about your choices? This is important to be able to make an informed decision about the role that would suit you, your skill set, and your experience best.

DOI: 10.4324/9781003542049-1

There are career routes within the broader field of psychology which are already quite clear and well known, for example, the role of a clinical psychologist. However, this book will help to layout in clear terms the newer PP roles and opportunities they offer.

Currently, it is not easy to find information on the roles together from one trusted source. This is because many of the developments for PP roles have happened quite separately. We are seeking to bring this information together in an easy-to-digest format that will allow for a clearer understanding for a wide audience.

With the recent introduction of registration for PPs via the British Psychological Society (BPS) and British Association of Behavioural and Cognitive Psychotherapies (BABCP), the profile of PP roles is continuing to be raised. Recent publications such as the *NHS Long Term Workforce Plan* (2023) have shown that psychological professions account for the biggest and fastest growth within the National Health Service (NHS) workforce. Within psychological professions, PPs now make up more than a quarter of that workforce. There have been further commitments made to training and growing the PP workforce over the coming years, so there is a need to ensure that those preparing to leave education, enter the workforce, and, in the early stages of their careers, understand the pathways into these roles.

How to Use This Book

We acknowledge that there are different ways in which you might access this book. This might depend on your reason for coming to it, for example, to find out more about a specific role you are interested in, or to gain an oversight of each of the PP roles as you determine where you would like your career to take you. It may also depend on your own reading preferences, if you are someone who prefers to read each chapter and move through the book cover to cover, or as someone who prefers to dip in and out, with an 'as needed' approach. We have therefore written this book with those varied needs in mind and hope that whichever approach you take you will find useful and inspiring information to digest.

This book includes chapters on each of the four PP roles individually – PWP, MHWP, CWP, and EMHP. Each of these chapters will include some background and outline the practitioner's role in detail, including but not limited to:

- information on the setting and specified system of care in which the practitioner operates;
- the population group supported;
- how the practitioner might undertake assessment and identify appropriate support;
- the evidence-based interventions the practitioner is trained to offer;
- other key aspects of working within the role.

With the newer roles of CWP, EMHP, and then MHWP being developed one after the other, as expansions and based on the success of the original PWP role, there are understandably areas of overlap in the information we give about each. We have purposely included these overlapping elements of information to allow each chapter to stand alone as an overview of the relevant role and to allow you to jump into a chapter of most interest without needing to have read through them in order.

To ensure that these role-specific chapters, and this overall book, bring to life the experience of being a PP, we have included a range of quotes and case examples. Quotes have been provided by those working in PP roles, those currently in training as PPs, those teaching them, providing their clinical supervision, employing them, and managing them in services. We have endeavoured to include a wide range of voices, across the range of practitioner roles and representing a range of backgrounds and identities. The authors will also draw on their own clinical experience to bring these chapters to life.

What we do need to acknowledge here is the identity and privilege of ourselves as authors, particularly as white women in a field overrepresented by this grouping. We have purposely reached out to others to try and broaden the range of experience shared. However, we also recognise and acknowledge the dominance of a white, 'Western' viewpoint in the field of psychology as a whole, including the evidence base we draw from as PPs and the interventions we offer, and support ongoing 'decolonising the curriculum' work and widening access initiatives across the United Kingdom.

As with the purposeful overlapping of information already mentioned, we may utilise quotes and input from PPs across more than one chapter. Again, this is holding in mind the way some of you may choose to read this book. We want to ensure that relevant quotes are included at key points rather than you needing to be redirected to a different chapter or potentially missing the opportunity for you to hear what real practitioners have to say.

Where we include real-life case examples of low-intensity, CBT-informed clinical practice, provided to us by real practitioners, we will not include that practitioner's name alongside the example. The practitioner remaining unnamed is our attempt to ensure the clients who are represented in these case examples maintain as much anonymity as possible. We will instead include the practitioners' names in our acknowledgements, to show appreciation for their contributions and in helping us bring the PP roles to life for you as readers.

Throughout this book, we will be talking to 'you', with our general assumption being that 'you' are someone who is either considering your options for a psychology informed career, already interested enough in a future career as a PP to have selected this book from the library or bookshop shelf in order to know more detail about the possible roles, or so interested in one of the roles as your next step in your career that you have already applied for or been accepted on a training programme. (If you have been accepted on a programme, then well done! Hopefully, this book will stoke your excitement for when you begin your training.)

We are also aware that there might be some reading this book who do not intend to pursue a career as a PP themselves. They may, instead, have picked up this book to get more insight into the roles of those they work alongside, adjacent to, or in leadership positions over. Or they may already be in one of the PP roles and want to know a little more about the 'sibling' PP roles, for example, a CWP or an EMHP who is curious about the PWP role that directly preceded them, a PWP or an MHWP who is curious about their counterparts working with children and YP (CWPs and EMHPs), or a PWP, a CWP, or an EMHP curious about the differences in the newest role on the block, the MHWP.

For this second grouping of people accessing this book, we acknowledge that the 'you' to whom we speak may not be a direct fit. However, we hope that this will still feel accessible to you and will give you the opportunity to learn about the roles, the ways in which they are similar and distinct, the ways in which they are being implemented around the country, and the careers that can be developed within each role.

One thing of which we, as authors and experienced PPs with several years under our belts in our respective PP roles (PWP for Elspeth and CWP for Kirsty), are particularly aware is how much we love our acronyms in this field of work! Already in this single paragraph, there have been three separate acronyms included. If you are new to this field, it may feel like a whole new language to learn. What we will do in this book, to support you in managing this, is include the full term on each first occasion of referring to something in a chapter that can be replaced with an acronym, with the acronym itself in brackets alongside it. Once this has been done, we will then use the acronym for the remainder of that chapter.

As you may have already seen, there is a handy acronym decoder included at the beginning of this book. This lists all the acronyms used within this book, as well as some additional acronyms that you may come across if you pursue a career or training in this field of work. We hope that you will be able to refer to this acronym decoder as needed to support your understanding.

In addition to this, we would like to add an explanation here in the introduction about our use of language throughout the chapters when referring to those people being supported by PPs. Some may call them service users, patients, or clients, in the world of adult working, and in the world of children and YP, those terms may be used as well as the words children, YP, adolescents, teenagers, and families to describe who is accessing support.

We have made the decision in our role-specific chapters to go with the most used term we have come across. For PWPs, we have gone with 'patients', whereas for MHWPs, we have used 'service users'. For CWPs and EMHPs, we have made use of the term 'young person' or 'young people', both being shortened to the acronym 'YP'. In the remaining chapters that cover multiple roles, we will generally use the term 'clients or young people', with the hopes that these choices are clear and inclusive.

Our Aim

What we hope, overall, is that by the time you reach the end of the chapter of particular interest to you, or the end of reading this book in full, you will have learned something new and gained a real sense of the PP roles. You will have heard from people who are excited about and dedicated to these roles, be they PPs themselves, their supervisors, managers, lecturers, and tutors, or us (Elspeth and Kirsty) as your authors. We certainly know that true passion for the roles is out there, as those we've spoken to have told us...

Laura Spence, a qualified CWP, tells us about her passion for the role, and particularly the training year.

> I am forever grateful for the opportunity the CWP training gave me. I have found a passion for clinical work and supporting YP at an early intervention level. This training has opened the doors for me to lots of other avenues for further professional development.

Eve Bampton-Wilton is a qualified PWP, senior lecturer, and clinical programme manager in the Psychological Professions Network. Eve spoke to us about her passion for these roles. She told us:

> As a PP, I think I thrive in my roles because I try to embody the principles of LICBT working in all the work that I do, staying motivated and enthusiastic and applying my CBT knowledge to what I do. I think my passion for the low-intensity role means I am a strong ally for PPs and am always thinking about developments in practice and how this applies to low-intensity.

Eve notes that, historically, more weight has been placed on other psychological roles. She says,

> I think speaking up and advocating for PPs helps with cultural change and building respect for our profession. This means the workforce can be better represented in the wider psychological professions. I think the practitioner workforce is diverse and PPs have a unique skillset that can help so many people. This, in turn, supports the increasingly diverse communities that we serve.

Elle Crane, a qualified CWP, HI CBT therapist, and clinical supervisor, tells us how she is anticipating publication of the book itself. She says,

> I'm genuinely excited to see this book take shape. Seeing the direct impact of the PP roles, as a CWP and then as a colleague and supervisor in Child and Adolescent Mental Health Service (CAMHS) teams and Mental Health Support Teams (MHSTs), I know the importance of these roles. This book will be incredibly valuable and a missing piece I have felt as a former CWP and a supervisor.

We hope to have inspired some excitement for building your own career as a PP, whichever role that may be in, and wish you the best for a rewarding and fulfilling experience.

Box 1.1   References and wider reading

British Association of Behavioural and Cognitive Psychotherapies (BABCP) website – https://babcp.com/
British Psychological Society (BPS) website – https://www.bps.org.uk/
NHS England. (2023). *NHS long term workforce plan*. NHS England.

Chapter 2

Being a Psychological Wellbeing Practitioner

Introduction

The Psychological Wellbeing Practitioner (PWP) role was the first of the psychological practitioner (PP) roles to be established. This chapter will take an in-depth look at the role from its inception to its current position and developments.

This chapter will explain what the PWP role involves, including assessment and treatment interventions, as well as learning about the different places where PWPs work.

The modalities in which treatment can be delivered will also be discussed, including computerised cognitive behavioural therapy (cCBT), groups, and one-to-one support, via telephone, online platforms, or face to face.

There will be a discussion of the stepped care model, its links to multidisciplinary team working, and the important role this plays in PWP work. The overview of the PWP role will be brought to life with examples of clinical work from practicing PWPs.

Background

In 2006, *The Depression Report: A New Deal for Depression and Anxiety Disorders* was published by Lord Layard and the Centre for Economic Performance Mental Health Policy Group. The report highlighted the major economic impact of anxiety and depression, through both reduced ability to work and increased reliance on benefits.

The report also highlighted that although National Institute for Health and Care Excellence (NICE) Guidelines clearly outline

DOI: 10.4324/9781003542049-2

effective treatments for these conditions, there was a shortage of trained therapists to deliver this evidence-based care.

Layard's report led to the development of the Improving Access to Psychological Therapies (IAPT) Programme. The economic rationale was clear; investing in training and providing evidence-based treatments would lead to fewer sickness absences and more people would be able to return to work, ultimately saving money in the long term.

In 2006, there were initially two pilot demonstration IAPT sites at Doncaster and Newham. Due to the success of the pilot sites, by 2008, the IAPT programme had been rolled out across England.

In 2023, following consultation, IAPT was renamed National Health Service (NHS) Talking Therapies for anxiety and depression (TTad). The aim of the rebrand was to improve public understanding of the remit of the services and the appropriateness of referrals in presentations of depression and anxiety disorders.

NHSTTad has been widely perceived to be successful and has been used to provide the foundation for similar mental health initiatives all over the world. Its ability to collect large amounts of data, including routine outcome measures, has contributed to its success (see 'Scope and Remit' below).

In order to ensure consistency in delivery, based on the evidence and data, NHS England (NHSE) produced the NHSTTad Manual. There have been several updates to the Manual with version 7 published in March 2024. Alongside this, there is the PWP curriculum, at the time of publication, the most recent update is the fourth edition, published in April 2023.

The data has also helped, alongside the NHS Long-Term Workforce Plan (LTWP), to secure commitment to funding for training and expansion of NHSTTad, including funding direct from the treasury, evidence of the recognised wider impact of NHSTTad on the economy, as well as health. The NHSE Operational Planning Guidance also continues to identify access to mental health services as a priority – a reassuring fact for those seeking a future career as a PWP.

Psychological professionals are the workforce group with the biggest expansion targets (LTWP), which is good news for those reading this book and considering a career in the psychological professions.

Scope and Remit

PWPs are trained to deliver brief low-intensity (LI) cognitive behavioural therapy (CBT)-based interventions for mild to moderate presentations of depression and anxiety disorders.

NHSTTad follows three key principles:

- Evidence-based treatment at an appropriate dose – NICE recommended treatment for the specific condition, at an intensity and duration that data shows will produce a clinical outcome
- Appropriately trained and supervised workforce that delivers high-quality interventions, with supervision, which ensures adherence to trained competencies. In addition, PWPs should be registered with the relevant professional body
- Routine outcome monitoring – the data component, supporting effective delivery clinically and operationally

The IAPT system was based on the stepped care model (see Figure 2.1). This model is designed to offer the least intrusive option first. At Step 1, watchful waiting and support are offered through the general practitioner (GP) and their practice staff.

NHSTTad work is delivered at Steps 2 and 3, with the PWP role sitting at Step 2. At Step 3, there are a variety of high-intensity

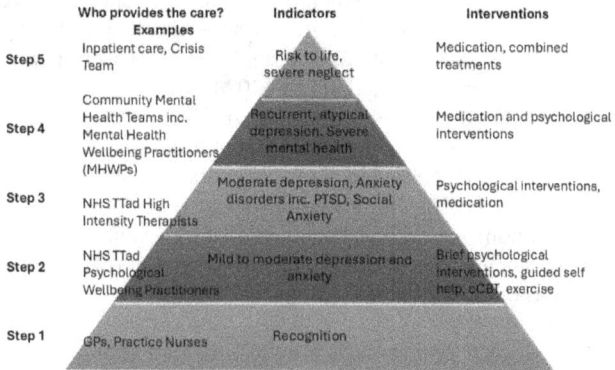

	Who provides the care? Examples	Indicators	Interventions
Step 5	Inpatient care, Crisis Team	Risk to life, severe neglect	Medication, combined treatments
Step 4	Community Mental Health Teams inc. Mental Health Wellbeing Practitioners (MHWPs)	Recurrent, atypical depression. Severe mental health	Medication and psychological interventions
Step 3	NHS TTad High Intensity Therapists	Moderate depression, Anxiety disorders inc. PTSD, Social Anxiety	Psychological interventions, medication
Step 2	NHS TTad Psychological Wellbeing Practitioners	Mild to moderate depression and anxiety	Brief psychological interventions, guided self help, cCBT, exercise
Step 1	GPs, Practice Nurses	Recognition	

Figure 2.1 The Stepped Care Model.

(HI) therapy roles, described in more detail in Chapter 14. Steps 4 and 5 are the focus of secondary care and inpatient services; they will include psychological professions but are outside the scope of practice for NHSTTad and therefore PWPs; however, NHSTTad may interface and refer into these Step 4 services and you may find Mental Health Wellbeing Practitioners (MHWPs) (Chapter 3) or some of the other roles discussed in Chapter 14 in these services.

PWPs provide Step 2 LI interventions through a case management model. This is a patient-centred approach, where the PWP assesses, provides intervention, and monitors outcomes, which are routinely discussed within the specified supervision structure. This consists of case management supervision (CMS) and clinical skills supervision (CSS) and is further described later in this chapter. PWP interventions are based on CBT models and principles and delivered through a guided self-help model, which includes psychoeducation.

PWPs are trained to treat mild to moderate depression and anxiety, including generalised anxiety disorder (GAD), panic disorder, and obsessive compulsive disorder (OCD). On average, PWPs will provide between four and six sessions as a dose of treatment.

PWPs are trained to deliver their interventions through a range of methods of delivery, including via telephone, face to face, and online platforms, for example, NHS Attend Anywhere. PWPs assess individuals and then treat patients on a one-to-one basis, as well as in groups and through cCBT.

PWP training is designed to support the development of skills in both 'common' and 'specific' therapeutic factors. Common factors explore the interpersonal communication skills required in patient contacts, such as developing rapport, active listening, and demonstrating empathy. These skills are key in ensuring PWPs gather information to achieve a shared understanding of the issues faced by their patients. Specific skills are those associated with the clinical interventions that PWPs are training in, for example, learning about specific interventions that are outlined below.

As well as being trained in specific interventions, PWPs undertake learning in equality, diversity, and inclusion, on their training course. Individual consideration of cultural competence and how to adapt practice to meet the needs of all patients is key, as high-lighted below by Vongai and covered further in Chapter 7.

> Personal circumstances and/or characteristics that I feel impact me in my role include being both young and Black. While much of my work is remote, I've found that my identity influences how I listen and interact with patients, especially when it comes to understanding the complexity of their lived experiences.
>
> I recognise that patients may bring their own cultural backgrounds, values, and beliefs into the sessions, and I aim to create a space where these are respected, even if they're not always explicitly addressed. Although much of my work is remote, I believe that my ability to remain open, non-judgemental, and sensitive to cultural nuances helps to establish trust. For patients from minority or underrepresented backgrounds, this can be particularly meaningful, as they may feel more understood or at ease, even if it's not something we directly discuss.
>
> Vongai Tepa, Qualified PWP

Traditionally, referrals to IAPT services were predominantly from GPs; however, in recent years, there has been the rapid development of additional pathways into services, including self-referral, now including in many service support from artificial intelligence (AI) technology.

PWPs are trained to, and will often, undertake the majority of assessments (sometimes referred to as Initial or Triage assessments) of the referrals into NHSTTad services. This first assessment in the service has an important function in assessing the patient's suitability for NHSTTad services, both in terms of presentation, risk, and readiness. For many, the PWP will help reach a shared decision about the correct pathway and treatment choice within NHSTTad; however, not everyone referred will present with a presentation to remain and be treated within NHSTTad. It is important for patients who won't be coming into NHSTTad, for PWPs to be able to appropriately identify other presenting needs, then refer or signpost on (provide information to the patient to help enable them to access an alternate form of support), before discharging from NHSTTad service.

As part of this assessment and then within the treatment process, the IAPT model incorporates the use of a Minimum Data Set (MDS) to support and guide assessment and treatment decisions. It also supports the monitoring of service outcomes (i.e., national targets). Data is collected using the following standardised routine outcome measures that make up the MDS:

Patient Health Questionnaire-9 (PHQ-9) – this is a brief, nine-item, screening measure for the presence and severity of depression symptoms.

Generalised Anxiety Disorder 7-item (GAD-7) – this is a brief, seven-item, screening measure to assess the frequency and severity of GAD symptoms.

Phobia Scale – this three-item scale assesses avoidance behaviours related to specific situations or objects.

Work and Social Adjustment Scale (WSAS) – this five-item scale helps consider the impact of mental health symptoms on the patient's level on function in relation to both work and social activities.

The MDS questionnaires have cutoffs for 'caseness'. The cutoffs are predefined scores on each measure and to be in 'caseness' means that the patient is scoring on, or above the cutoff; therefore, indicating that the symptoms the patient is experiencing, when measures are first used at assessment, meet the threshold requiring intervention within NHSTTad.

The measures are then also used session by session. The PWP will reflect on the scores with the patient and use measures to support the monitoring of progress, directly in session and in Caseload Management Supervision with their supervisor. As the intervention progresses, the MDS cutoffs are also used to monitor whether a patient has moved into recovery (out of caseness) or has reliably improved (scores have improved significantly but not taken the patient out of caseness). All MDS data is collated and published nationally to support learning and accountability.

As well as the developments in pathways into NHSTTad, there have also been advances in digital therapy offers, such as cCBT packages supported by PWPs. Both self-referral and cCBT approaches have been further developed through the use of AI-assisted technologies. These developments have seen the advent of chatbots that can assist in triage of patients, as well as programmes of online materials: this is an area that is likely to see significant investment and change over the next few years, as the technologies are refined. There is evidence of these progressions in the use of digital technology accelerating, already following the impact of the COVID-19 pandemic, when services had to adapt to respond to restrictions in traditional face-to-face delivery. During that period, there was a significant increase in the uptake of digital technology, particularly in the use of telephone and online modalities and platforms to conduct assessments and deliver groups.

Population Served and Specified Systems of Care

Originally created for working-age adults in primary care but has since been developed to also support those in forensic services, older people, and patients with long-term conditions (LTCs) (National Collaborating Centre for Mental Health, 2018).

PWPs are able to deliver interventions that meet the needs of adults with mild to moderate depression and anxiety disorders (GAD, panic disorder, OCD, and support where sleep is impacted).

The PWP role is designed to meet the needs of adults, though local commissioning arrangements mean that some services may be commissioned to take patients from 16+, where others do not take until 18+.

To work as a registered PWP, a qualified practitioner needs to work within a specified system of care. For PWPs, this means that their service needs to have the ability to step up (i.e., secondary care) and down (i.e., to GP) according to patient need, and there should be clear and appropriate pathways of care. Services PWPs work in should also have good clinical governance procedures (accountability for the delivery of safe, high-quality care).

Though the PWP role can exist in a variety of settings, most commonly PWPs will be found within specific NHSTTad; however, there are also NHS Commissioned Services, including TTad, delivered by the voluntary community and social enterprise sector partners, and PWPs can also be found working and delivering interventions within the Prison System.

A developing area of practice in NHSTTad is pathways for people with long-term physical health conditions and medically unexplained symptoms. There has been the development of guidance and the launch of the LTC Top-Up Training for PWPs. More recent work has also highlighted the importance of these developments, such as the Psychological Professions Network (PPN) Psychological Practice in Physical Health Discussion Paper. The development of the work of PWPs with patients with LTCs varies depending on a variety of factors but includes co-located services, physical health condition-specific pathways, and specifically designed groups and courses.

Supervision

Key to the safe and effective implementation and management of this high-volume role are CMS and CSS. Supervision supports fidelity to the evidence base, case management, clinical governance, skills development, and general support of the PWPs' wellbeing.

CMS is patient-focused and ensures that the patient is receiving the most appropriate care. It is one hour weekly, individual supervision, usually with a Senior PWP (SPWP). It allows an opportunity for the regular review of the full caseload. PWPs are required to bring all new cases, cases with risk concerns and MDS scores above predetermined thresholds, and all cases should be reviewed at no more than four weekly time points. CMS ensures fidelity to the LI treatment model, as well as an opportunity for PWPs to seek further support or advice.

CSS is more PWP-focused and ensures that they are maintaining the required level of knowledge and skill for their role. CSS can be delivered in groups. It is a structured process with a clinician knowledgeable in the LI model and interventions. It allows discussion of cases in more depth, including guidance and feedback that also support the PWP in developing and consolidating their skills and ensuring that work is safe and within the PWP scope of practice.

Both CMS and CSS are essential to the effective and safe practice of PWPs, for the benefit of patients but also for the wellbeing of the PWP.

The supervisor should have a minimum of one year's post-qualification experience, but it is recommended that it should ideally be at least two years. The supervisor should be competent in both the delivery of LI supervision and in the LI interventions they are supervising.

Pre-Intervention

As we move to begin to discuss the clinical work PWPs complete on a day-to-day basis, we take a moment to reflect on the PWPs LI CBT model and its impact:

> I wanted to support people recover from depression and anxiety, and I believed Low Intensity CBT could help people do that. Over a decade later, I still believe that. I am very grateful to continue to be able to work with individuals to help them to a better place in their life.
>
> Sam Torney, NHS TT Team Lead

In many NHSTTad services, PWPs complete the majority of assessments. Assessments are completed at the point at which an individual is coming into a service and help to ascertain whether that individual is appropriate for that talking therapy service. It may be that the individual is appropriate for a PWP to support, or it may be that the triage assessment indicates that they are either suitable for another step of the talking therapy service or not suitable and need to be referred either onwards or outwards from the talking therapy service. Depending on the local commissioning arrangements, this could be into or out of the NHS.

The PWP curriculum trains PWPs to assess in a patient-centred way. Considering the patient's presenting problem, their current symptoms, and the impact these are having, as well as any risk (see below) before discussing how the service may be able to meet the patient's needs in a collaborative way.

In this section, we will focus more on initial assessment, but just before we do, it is important to consider risk assessment.

Risk assessment occurs within both triage and initial assessments, but also at many other points within the patients care journey. There is the need to risk assess to ensure that the patient receives appropriate care and support. This could be a topic of several books in its own right, and therefore, this is only a very brief overview of the topic.

It is important not to be afraid of asking questions in terms of risk assessment; research shows that asking about suicide does not increase the risk of patients acting on these thoughts. There are ways in which PWPs can approach this topic and build rapport with the patient, to ask the right questions at the right time, making them supportive, meaningful, and protective for the patient. Many services use a 5Ps framework, covering presenting problem, predisposing factors, precipitating factors, perpetuating factors, and protective factors. Once this information is gathered, a PWP, with the support of CMS, works to consider the best treatment option for the patient and can work with the patient to create a safety plan.

In April 2025, NHSE published 'Staying safe from suicide'; this guidance co-produced with patient and public voice promotes a person-centred approach with a focus on understanding a person's situation and managing safety.

An initial assessment with the patient at the point at which the PWP is taking that patient on specifically to their LI caseload to deliver a PWP-specific LI CBT-based intervention will be problem-focused. Here, we begin to introduce some of the models that support PWPs in their work. A five areas model is based on CBT principles. The model can be used to gather information about the patient's presentation in the key areas.

In Figure 2.2, you're looking at a five areas model, which contains the four factors that make up the individual, so you

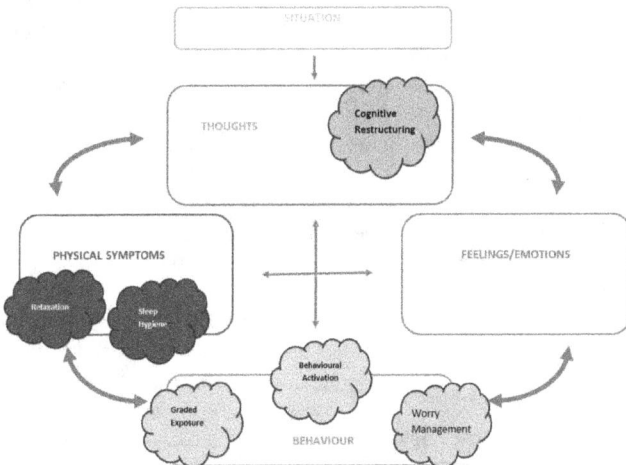

Figure 2.2 The Five Areas Model.

have got your thoughts, feelings, physical symptoms, and behaviours. At the top, you've got your situational factors, most often external to the individual. This can be a really insightful model to use with patients to help them see how these areas interact and impact upon each other (the arrows). It helps to support the identification of vicious cycles that are part of the maintenance of the patient's symptoms. For example, an avoidance behaviour or a negative automatic thought (NAT) can maintain a feeling of low mood.

It is also a useful model to help identify particular interventions that would help break a patient's vicious cycles and help build some virtuous cycles. These can be seen in the clouds in Figure 2.2, and each intervention is discussed in more detail below.

PWPs also utilise the 'COM-B' model, which is grounded in behaviour change theory. This model has three key factors: Capability (C), Opportunity (O), and Motivation (M), all of which influence a person's Behaviour (B).

Within the initial assessment, the PWP is exploring a patient's symptoms with them to begin to formulate their difficulties and using a shared understanding to develop a 'Problem Statement'. The problem statement makes clear the issue that will be the focus of the LI intervention. The PWP is looking to, in a patient-centred way, come to a point of shared decision-making about the next steps in support and which intervention will be most appropriate for the problem identified. The problem statement then becomes a point of focus during intervention to ensure that you're meeting and continue to meet the patient's needs as the intervention progresses.

Signposting is a key aspect of the PWP role. As practitioners deliver LI interventions to high volumes of patients in a time-limited format, it is not possible or appropriate to do everything!

Signposting could be seen as an intervention; in fact, in the Reach Out Manual, it is classed as one. It can be utilised through the treatment process; however, in practice, it is often used, for example, at the end of an assessment, and therefore, it feels appropriate to describe it here in the Pre-Intervention section: particularly as there may be patients seen for assessment who don't move on to have PWP Intervention but who may benefit from some tailored signposting.

So what is signposting, and how can it be done well in practice?

Signposting can refer to a range of resources, including literature, local social groups, specialist counselling services, or food banks. There are far too many options to list, and these will vary between areas and regions.

That is why knowing your local area is key. It is also important to have an understanding of the quality and relevance of services you may signpost to, and some questions you could ask yourself are as follows:

Who are your local population?

What are their specific needs?

What is available in your area?

Are the services able and appropriately qualified to offer the services they advertise?

Is it free or low cost?

Finally, how do you and your service update and review knowledge of local services, particularly as there are often funding changes, other financial pressures, or criteria changes, even, waiting list closures that impact on the delivery of services in the community.

Interventions

My favourite thing about my role is seeing the difference in someone from the start of their sessions to the end. Seeing how far someone has come and seeing their hard work paying off. PWPs do a great job of giving people the information and techniques to manage their symptoms while promoting independence.

Kelly DeSantis, PWP

PWP treatments consist of a range of LI CBT-informed evidence-based interventions delivered through a remit of guided self-help. These PWP interventions can be delivered in a one-to-one format, face to face, via telephone or video platform, with the intervention provided tailored specifically to the presentation and goals of the patient; however, many services also have other modes of delivery.

Groups

These include the development and utilisation of groups to deliver their Step 2 PWP-led interventions. These groups can vary in size, from small rooms to lecture-style delivery. Groups are usually led by two PWPs with the support of PowerPoint slides or other supporting materials, that is, Booklets. Groups at Step 2 are delivered as educational style groups and not group therapy. They can be delivered face to face or via video platforms.

Computerised Cognitive Behavioural Therapy

If a service offers cCBT, PWPs are often the practitioners delivering the associated support. NICE Guidelines recommend that cCBT is most effective if it is supported by a trained practitioner. There are a number of providers of cCBT therapy programmes and packages. An NHSTTad service will consider their, and their populations, needs and requirements and often externally commission a provider. These cCBT packages host large databases of psychoeducation and guided self-help materials. They have interactive components, and the patient receives a login to access and work through these materials in their own time and pace. The PWP opens access to relevant materials, reviews, and supports alongside the package, often via email message or brief telephone contacts.

Whether through 1:1, group, or cCBT, PWPs are trained to utilise specific LI interventions, and there is also an expectation of the patient completing between-session tasks at home. These tasks are designed to support the patient in becoming their own therapist and developing a toolkit of interventions that they can continue to use, even after their sessions with the PWP have ended.

Psychoeducation

Throughout these interventions, and indeed this chapter, there is reference to psychoeducation. Psychoeducation refers to the information and support provided to patients to help them better understand and cope with their difficulties. The power of this component is often undervalued, but this should not be the case, and PWPs can and should use it meaningfully as a key part of intervention in their practice, to help empower their patients.

Below is a brief summary of the core PWP interventions.

Behavioural Activation

Behavioural activation (BA) is an intervention based on the behavioural theory of depression. BA is an intervention that helps the patient address reductions in activity levels that maintain their depression. BA is considered a stand-alone treatment; however, it is also a component intervention of HI CBT treatment. There is substantial evidence base supporting the effectiveness of BA, with research showing that the LI delivery of BA can be as effective as its use within a broader HI CBT treatment.

BA aims to target avoidance and re-establish routine in patients experiencing symptoms of low mood or depression. Depression is often associated with a reduction in activity; however, BA also considers persons who are managing to function in regard to routine activity but may be lacking in a particular kind of activity, that is, pleasurable activity, or where the activities they are undertaking do not match or meet their values.

Therefore, in this intervention, it is important to consider routine, necessary, and pleasurable activities. A PWP will often begin by establishing a baseline diary of routine. This diary can be used between sessions as a homework task. The PWP and the patient can then review the information brought back to the session by the patient, allowing for curious conversations and beginning to develop a hierarchy of activity. Before planning the introduction of activity back into the patient's diary, a common feature that is utilised in the planning of new activity is increasing activity that is in line with the patient's values, or the things that matter to them.

Once new activities are introduced, the PWP will support the patient across a number of sessions to reflect on how this impacts their mood, consider building on the activities, and plan for increasing activity further going forward in a balanced way.

Below is an example of how Nick incorporates Values-Based Behavioural Activation into his practice in an NHSTTad practice with patients with an LTC:

> When working alongside patients who are significantly impacted by long-term health conditions, Values Based Behavioural Activation is an incredible intervention. It focuses on supporting patients in attaining purpose, meaning, fulfilment and quality in their day to day lives. The reason why I find it effective with LTCs is that if focuses less on "what can I not do" and more on "what aspects of my life do I value and what can I do to ensure these areas are being met". I find this helps the patient to alter their perspective and supports them in being creative and curious in what they are capable of doing in areas that are valuable to them. I find with Values Based BA there is a deeper level of engagement with patients who may be somewhat restricted by traditional Behavioural Activation due to aspects of mobility, pain and fatigue.
>
> Nick Jackson, Senior PWP

Graded Exposure

Graded Exposure (GE) is an intervention that can be offered by PWPs for anxiety presentations where avoidance is a key factor in keeping the problem going (maintenance of the problem).

The avoidance of situations and or objects due to fear only provides short-term relief from the anxiety symptoms, and longer term is a maintaining factor. GE is the planned therapeutic confrontation to a feared situation, object, or memory. The GE intervention is based on supporting the patient to have gradually increasing amounts of contact with the object or situation causing anxiety.

There are four factors important to the successful implementation of the GE intervention:

1   Grading – of the stimuli, for example, pictures moving onto real objects
2   Prolonged – enough time for the anxiety symptoms to reduce (at least a 50% reduction) in the presence of situation or object
3   Repeated – it is not enough to do the task once

4 Without distraction – the individual must experience a level of fear to be able to notice the reduction

The PWP begins by supporting the patient to create a hierarchy. Then, starting with the least anxiety-provoking, plan with the patient to begin the Exposure tasks, usually as between-session activities, with the patient remaining in the situation until they experience habituation.

For an example of GE in practice, see 'Managing Panic' below.

Exposure Response Prevention

Exposure Response Prevention (ERP) is an LI intervention that can be used in the treatment of mild OCD. Obsessions can be in the form of thoughts, images, impulses, or urges experienced by the individual, which cause significant anxiety and distress. The compulsions are the actions the individual takes to reduce distress (i.e., excessive handwashing, checking, ordering/arranging, counting, and seeking reassurance).

In ERP, the PWP is looking to support gradual exposure to the anxiety-provoking triggers that cause the obsessions, without engaging in the compulsions.

ERP is designed to help patients manage their symptoms and therefore reduce avoidance and reassurance seeking.

It is best practice for a PWP to complete ERP with a patient under the supervision of someone trained to deliver CBT for OCD, to support the planning and grading of the intervention.

Cognitive Restructuring

We need to ensure competence across all the interventions and work collaboratively with the patient using shared decision-making, but you may find, as Vongai describes below, that you have an intervention that resonates more with you as a PP:

> For me, my favourite core step two intervention is Cognitive Restructuring (CR). I really connect with the psychoeducation with CR, I think it almost creates 'lightbulb' moments for patient s. I love the grittiness of explaining more about how these thoughts are formed and patterns created. Once we get

through to the actual thought challenging, it's like 'lightbulbs' again because patients realise there is not as much factual evidence for their thoughts as perhaps they felt at the time. I find CR to be one of the most empowering interventions, because at its core it is reminding patients that how they speak to others, is also how they should speak to themselves.

Marin Cash, Qualified PWP

Thoughts are a major component of many of the presentations of patients seeking support for their mental health (depression and anxiety), as referenced as a part of the five areas model above. These NATs or 'unhelpful thoughts' can act as a powerful maintaining factor for the patient.

The role of PWPs is to support the patient in challenging these unhelpful thoughts. This is first done by identifying the thoughts on a thought record and, in particular, the 'hot thought' (most related to the emotion). There is then the process of looking for evidence for and against the thought before reconsidering the thought.

Unhelpful thoughts can occur in both low mood and anxiety presentations; here, Vongai demonstrates the application of Cognitive Restructuring (CR) in an anxiety presentation:

Cognitive restructuring is a useful and beneficial intervention because it helps patients start to understand and break the cycle of unhelpful thinking, particularly in anxiety-provoking situations. By identifying negative thought patterns, we can pinpoint their triggers and replace them with more balanced, realistic thoughts.

What I like about the cognitive restructuring intervention is that it often leads to a 'light bulb' moment for patients. When they realise how quickly their mind jumps to the worst-case scenarios, it's like a weight lifts. I find that they start to see how their thoughts, feelings, and behaviours are all connected, and it suddenly feels possible to make a change.

In my work as a PWP, I have been able to use the Cognitive Restructuring intervention to help with problems such as anxiety, where patients tend to catastrophise situations. Helping them recognise their automatic negative thoughts allows us to identify the source of emotional distress and consider perspectives that are more helpful and balanced.

One example is when I worked with a patient who was anxious about meeting work deadlines. She often thought, "I'm going to fail and disappoint everyone, and I'll lose my job." Using CR, we examined the evidence behind this thought and explored more balanced alternatives. By doing this, she realised that her anxiety was based on assumptions rather than facts, and this helped her feel more confident in managing her workload.

Vongai Tepa, Qualified PWP

Managing Panic

Panic disorder is a catastrophic misinterpretation of physical symptoms and fear of consequences. It is where an individual has recurrent or unexpected panic attacks, leading to behaviour change, avoidance, and/or attempts to prevent panic attacks, including safety behaviours.

Panic disorder requires the PWP to gather information; this can be done utilising a panic diary. Following on from this is the psychoeducation phase, including information about the fight-flight response (the body's physiological response to perceive threat or danger). PWPs can utilise two of their LI interventions with patients to support them in developing a toolkit to manage their panic disorder: GE and CR.

Here Nick talks us through how he utilises GE with a patient experiencing panic disorder and how the benefits of learning the technique in sessions can have lasting benefits:

I find Graded Exposure to be a hugely valuable intervention when working with patients who experience Panic Disorder, especially where specific environments, activities or situations are available for the patient to confront reliably. The reason I find it works so well is it allows patients to face and overcome their fears by gradually exposing themselves to manageable levels of anxiety which can in turn feel more achievable. Overtime it helps the patient in reducing the intensity of their responses through repetition and habituation, therein, increasing their tolerance to the feared activity or situation. I really like that it provides a framework that is easy for the patient to follow which is controlled, measured and can be replicated to support their onward journey outside of therapy. Aside from the obvious benefits of supporting patients in overcoming and facing their anxiety. It is one of the interventions that I feel has a much wider range of benefits, such as increased self-esteem, confidence, an increased sense of achievement and control.

Nick Jackson, Senior PWP

Behavioural Experiments

Behavioural Experiments (BEs) are structured activities that can be used to test the validity of negative thoughts. The thought to be tested is identified, along with the person's predicted outcomes. A plan is then developed to test these predictions. The PWP can also support the patient to identify any potential barriers and ideas for how these may be overcome.

Paul Thompson, PWP Course Lecturer, provides an example here for consideration. Firstly, where an individual has a thought that they cannot achieve a specific activity and this is leading to inactivity and low mood. The BE process can identify the thought ("I can't do anything productive, so there's no point even trying."), with a cognitive hypothesis of "If I try to engage in a small, manageable activity, I'll fail or it won't help." The PWP and patient can then work to develop an activity that tests this negative assumption. "The experiment tests the accuracy of their negative predictions and demonstrates the potential mood-lifting and motivational effects of engaging in small, achievable tasks, ultimately reducing behavioural avoidance and inactivity associated with depression." Successful completion of the activity supports the build-up of evidence that the thought is inaccurate.

A different application of BEs within a panic disorder scenario where GE was not appropriate, demonstrates the importance of considering the individual patient and the ability of the PWP to tailor their toolkit and support the patient:

I really enjoy using Behavioural Experiments in conjunction with Interoceptive Exposure, especially when working with patients experiencing panic disorder where Graded Exposure is not a viable option. This tends to be the case when the patient's presenting panic does not lend itself well to a specific environment or where the fear of experiencing physical symptoms of panic is more pervasive. For example, those with predictions of experiencing a panic attack in an environment where repetition cannot be achieved, panic that occurs "out of the blue" or without apparent trigger.

Conducting Behavioural Experiments with the support of appropriate clinical supervision can be a wonderful way to support the patient in challenging and testing out their prediction or belief that experiencing physical symptoms of panic, for example, will cause them to lose control, faint or that something bad is going to happen to them. I likewise find it to be helpful to have a specific framework which allows the patient to reflect on their experience in a helpful and positive light. Objectively, I notice that using Behavioural Experiments with Interoceptive Exposure significantly reduces the need to undertake additional interventions such as Cognitive Restructuring, as it is a way of testing out their beliefs in real time and within a safe/controlled environment.

Nick Jackson, Senior PWP

Worry Management

Worry management is a useful and beneficial intervention because it helps people take back some control over their worries and puts them back in the driver's seat. As a PWP, I like worry management because it can be explained really easily and logically it makes sense.

I use worry management a lot, especially in my work with patients with LTCs, where their physical health is impacting their mental health and they have tests, hospital appointments or if they are dealing with a lot of uncertainty.

Kelly DeSantis, Qualified PWP

Worry is frequently a feature of GAD. Where this worry is identified as problematic for the patient, PWPs can offer a worry management (WM) intervention. This intervention is behavioural in nature and can be particularly useful for helping a patient where the *act* (or behaviour) of worrying is the main thing that is getting in the way of day-to-day life and the things the patient would rather be doing.

Supporting the patient to identify the type of worry they are experiencing is one of the first steps in WM. The types of worry are generally categorised as 'real' or 'hypothetical'.

Once the patient understands the two different types of worry, they can practice sorting their worries. A 'Worry Tree' can be a helpful resource to give patients to support them with this.

There are then different ways of dealing with each type of worry. If the worry is 'real', then the PWP can introduce the problem-solving technique as a strategy to utilise to manage the problem underlying and causing the worry (see problem-solving intervention below).

If the worry is 'hypothetical' (or a 'what if worry'), then the patient is supported to recognise this and understand that there isn't anything they can do to change whether the worry will happen or not. They can then make use of 'let it go' techniques to take their mind off the worry. The PWP may spend time helping the patient develop their own range of 'let it go' techniques, finding out what is most helpful for them.

Where the worry is impacting on the process of engaging in other activities, 'Worry Time' can also be a practical strategy to teach. This is where a patient sets aside a specific time to focus on worry. Noting worries as they arise during other times but not engaging with them until the specified 'worry time'. This can give the patient a different perspective on their worries. In addition, they can ensure that they set the 'worry time' period at a time when they feel more able to implement the other WM strategies.

Here, Sheldon describes the process and benefits he finds in practice for himself and his patients when implementing the WM strategies:

> The conversational use of 'don't worry' is somewhat prevalent. Now whilst worries can serve some functional benefits, such as supporting us planning ahead and being prepared for situations, excessive worrying can be a product of and trigger for anxiety. Many patients report that the pervasive nature of unmanaged worry can disrupt various areas of their lives, such as work, relationships, sleep, and cognitive functioning. However, through scheduling a dedicated period daily to engage with and reflect on worries only, through 'Worry Time',

patient s can learn their current patterns of worry in thinking and behaviour, and gain self-governance on how to contain their worry, and associated anxiety. This strategic intervention for worry management, is rewarding for me to support patients with. As is the goal, patients report finding it beneficial setting boundaries with their time, where they can address important worries that cause distress, but also spend time for themselves and be able to function efficiently in day-to-day life. With a refined sense of control on worrying habits, patients find they have more time for self-care, being present when with loves ones, engaging better with responsibilities, and/or seeing the future more positively, which is greatly satisfying to acknowledge as a practitioner.

Sheldon Rodrigues, Senior PWP

Problem-Solving

Problem-solving is a practical approach that PWPs can teach to patients, particularly if there are practical or situational factors impacting on their low mood or anxiety.

The role of PWPs is not to solve the patient's problem(s) for them but to teach them the seven-step problem-solving approach, as a strategy, to allow the patient to gain the skill in their toolkit to solve their problems, particularly when problems are identified by the patient as being too big to solve, initially.

The problem-solving approach works through a seven-step process, and it can be beneficial to encourage the patient to write down notes to help them work through the steps in a systematic way and to help them gain some additional clarity that may be more challenging if they are anxious, low, or worrying, and this is impacting on their thought processes.

The steps are outlined below:

1 Identify the problem
2 Identify the solution
3 Analyse strengths and weaknesses
4 Select a solution
5 Plan implementation
6 Implementation
7 Review

It may initially appear straightforward, especially if you yourself are not feeling low or anxious, but it can be a powerful intervention to add to someone's toolkit in practice:

> Sometimes we can feel so overwhelmed by anxious thoughts that we cannot think of a way to solve the problems we are facing. Problem Solving helps to break down the problems step by step to create suitable solutions. The Problem Solving intervention is very simplistic but effective.
>
> Kelly DeSantis, Qualified PWP

Promoting Good Sleep

Good-quality sleep is a key foundation to mental and physical wellbeing; conversely, poor sleep can be the result of, or contribute to, poor physical and mental wellbeing. When completing an assessment with a patient, questions around sleep will be part of the assessment; there is also a question in the PHQ-9. It is important to consider both the amount and quality of the sleep a patient is getting. This can be done by utilising a sleep diary as a between-session task, as well as by using questions and MDS. Diaries may help not only to establish patterns and triggers but also to monitor progress with the intervention.

Sleep difficulties are often a factor in both anxiety and depression presentations. Changes and improvements to achieve more restful and effective sleep can be beneficial both for symptoms and enable patients to feel more resourced to engage in interventions. It can be a good foundation to complete with patients for whom a step up may be required.

The intervention itself can include psychoeducation on normal sleep and factors that may impact on this. Followed by further consideration of factors in practice and establishing regular sleep routines.

Physical Activity and Medication

Promoting physical activity is not a CBT-based approach; however, given the close associations between physical and mental health, this is an area PWPs may find of benefit to their patients. There are also links between promoting physical activity and the

BA intervention; however, it is not just getting a patient to join a gym!

For example, PWPs could deliver a psychoeducational course covering skills for wellbeing, including interventions such as BA and CR with a physical activity element. Where the physical element, such as a walk or stretching (with an appropriately qualified individual), is included as part of the session time each week.

Many areas now also have connections with exercise referral schemes or pathways with physical activity providers. With new guidance produced in April 2024, 'Incorporating physical activity interventions into NHS Talking Therapies A toolkit' further supporting the development of this work.

Although medication adherence in itself is not a CBT-based approach, given the large numbers of patients prescribed or considering medication as part of their treatment plan, it is important for PWPs to be aware of the pharmacological treatments for anxiety and depression.

It is very important to be very clear with patients the boundaries and limitations of this advice. PWPs are not medical professionals or prescribers; however, being able to gather information, for example, on non-concordance can open up helpful communication – allowing the PWP to give accurate information about antidepressants, for example, that it can take a number of weeks at a therapeutic dose before beneficial effects are observed.

The PWP can also work collaboratively with a patient in order to make shared decisions about what to do next if a patient has concerns regarding their medication. These options could include the patient arranging a medication review with the GP, to the PWP completing a more detailed risk assessment, depending on the nature of the information discussed and disclosed.

Qualification, Agenda for Change, and Registration

The PWP qualification can now be taken at a level 6 or 7, as an undergraduate or postgraduate route (but training centres may not offer all routes).

There is also the level 6 apprenticeship route to becoming a PWP. For this, there is the requirement that an English and mathematics qualification to level 2 must be achieved. If you do not have this at the beginning of training, you must undertake this 'functional skills qualification' alongside the PWP work. The apprenticeship route is intended for people without a degree but who have relevant life experience.

All of the routes, with British Psychological Society (BPS) course accreditation, lead to a PWP qualification at either Grad-Cert or PGCert, depending on the entry route.

More information on routes into the profession is covered in Chapter 6.

Agenda for Change

Agenda for Change (AfC) is the NHS pay system, which was introduced to standardise pay and conditions for NHS workers. Those PWPs within NHSTTad services will be paid on AfC Bands. For trainees, this is AfC Band 4, and once qualified, PWPs are paid at AfC Band 5. PWPs employed in other non-NHS organisations may have slightly different pay and conditions of employment.

Registration

PWP Registration became mandated in June 2022. PWPs can register with either the BPS or the British Association of Behavioural and Cognitive Psychotherapies.

In order to register, PWPs need to have completed a BPS-accredited PWP course. More information on gaining and maintaining Registration is covered in Chapter 9, Professional Ethics, and Chapter 11, Starting Out.

Developing Within and Beyond the PWP Role

Since the initial inception and rollout of the PWP role, the landscape has changed considerably. However, the PWP role can, and should, be considered to be a destination career and valued in its own right. That said, the role of the PWP has now also developed a potential career pathway beyond its original design. There are now lots of options for PWPs to progress and develop using their skills as a base. Other chapters within this book will go into these areas in much more detail, but it is important that we consider them here so that you know which chapters to go to, to look for different pieces of information.

Chapter 11 will look at the first-year post-qualification, starting out working in a psychological practitioner role, including registration, consolidation of learning and skills, and building a caseload.

Chapter 12 will explore making the most out of your career. For those with an interest in progressing, there is a discussion of potential training opportunities that are available for developing supervisory skills (CLM and CSS). There are also other training opportunities, such as LTC training, which is recommended to be completed within two years post-qualification. Chapter 12 will also consider *Becoming a Senior* and options such as taking on a *Champion Role*.

Whilst keen to promote the value of the PWP role in its own right, we also acknowledge some will seek further development within their career. Chapter 13 is where some of these options will be explored, considering the *Clinical Leadership, Operational, Teaching,* and *Research* options.

But just to give an overview and summary of the options now available, we are going to talk about them briefly here. One of the first things to consider when you are looking to progress and develop within a role is whether you want that to be a clinical pathway development or a more operational pathway of development. With a clinical pathway, you will remain working with patients, though this may become less direct, and through more supervisory or from clinical advisory roles. This may involve clinical guidance, but the work will remain very patient-focused.

With the more clinical development route, you might first want to consider developing your supervisory skills, for example, in the direction of caseload management, supporting trainees coming into service. Thinking about putting yourself forward for supervisor training will require conversations with your Line Manager, usually through discussion in your professional development reviews. If you complete supervisor training, you may then look to move to begin to deliver CLM and CSS to PWPs with less experience in yourself, before perhaps, looking to take on a SPWP role.

Becoming a SPWP involves taking on some of the additional tasks that this role encompasses, and a lot of these will depend on the service that you're in and how that's set up and exactly what the senior job description and personal specification requires. It is always worth checking with your service and in your areas to see what the SPWP looks like.

There are now clinical opportunities for PWPs to progress further with their clinical leadership, taking roles, such as Deputy Clinical Lead and Step 2 Clinical Lead roles within NHSTTad services or equivalents, with the associated increases in salary.

One of the other options, if you're not interested in clinical leadership, but still wish to develop clinically, are specialist PWP roles, for example, LTC Pathway developments. This route could begin with an informal champion role in an area of particular interest to you. NHSTTad has some specifically identified champion roles (including Veterans and Perinatal), but some services also have additional roles developed based on local need.

A champion role is an excellent opportunity if you've got a passion about a particular subject area and you know it's one that you are keen to promote, develop, and support your colleagues and staff with, for the benefit of patients.

Following the operational route, you are moving into managerial aspects, service data, and targets. There will also be the development of skills in people management as well. That's where thinking about transferable skills from Chapter 7 might come in, because there are lots of skills within the PWP role that can help you move towards the more operational management, because you're still working and dealing with people regularly. In terms of the operational roles, these may include deputy team leads, team leads, or service managers within NHSTTad services.

There are also other options for development within the academic realm, teaching, and research. Many PWPs are now involved in training the next generation of PPs. There has also been a lot more developed recently in terms of growing the evidence base, through research at universities and in service, for example, Quality Improvement Projects. Throughout all the PP roles, we talk about the evidence-based practice that we do, and there's a lot of research that's been done in terms of the roles we do, what interventions we do and could be doing, but for now, it's about developing and progressing that field further.

The research element of the role might begin with something in service if you're able to see a particular need or opportunity. If this need or opportunity can be explored and developed, you may be able to write it up as part of an internal quality improvement project or look to see if you can approach one of the publications that publish LI work to share it on a wider platform. There are also other opportunities; for example, the PPNs have a newsletter for sharing information. The PPN North West PPs Community of Practice Newsletter is a localised example of where you can be supported to develop and share event reports, case studies, and so on, so it's again looking at what's available in your local area which allows you to develop these skills. This may be a personal interest initially, but the more that we develop our research and understanding as PPs, that also how we grow and support our profession and its evidence base.

Conclusion

We hope that this chapter has given you a good insight into the PWP role and what this can look like in practice. Is this the PP role for you?

If not, please visit Chapter 3 to learn about the other adult practitioner role, MHWP, or Chapters 4 and 5 to explore the children and young people's practitioner roles, the CWP and EMHP.

If the PWP role does sound like a good fit, then that's wonderful and welcome to NHSTTad – you may want to move on to Chapter 6 and beyond to continue exploring your career options.

Box 2.1   References and wider reading

Layard, R., Clark, D., Bell, S., Knapp, M., Meacher, B., & Priebe, S. (2006). *The depression report: A new deal for depression and anxiety disorders*. The Centre for Economic Performance's Mental Health Policy Group. London School of Economics. https://eprints.lse.ac.uk/818/1/DEPRESSION_REPORT_LAYARD.pdf

National Collaborating Centre for Mental Health. (2018). *The improving access to psychological therapies (IAPT) pathway for people with long-term physical health conditions and medically unexplained symptoms: Full implementation guidance.* National Collaborating Centre for Mental Health.

NHS England. (2023). *NHS long term workforce plan.* NHS England.

NHS England. (2023). *National curriculum for psychological wellbeing practitioner (PWP) programmes. V.4.3.* NHS England.

NHS England. (2024). *NHS talking therapies for anxiety and depression manual. 7th Edition.* NHS England. https://www.england.nhs.uk/wp-content/uploads/2018/06/nhs-talking-therapies-manual-v7.1-updated.pdf

NHS England. (2025). *Staying safe from suicide.* NHS England.

Psychological Professions Network. (2023). *Psychological practice in physical health: Discussion paper.* PPN. https://www.ppn.nhs.uk/resources-url/ppn-publications/470-ppn-discussion-paper-psychological-practice-in-physical-health-fv1-1-nov-2023/file

Richards, D.A., & Whyte, M. (2011). *Reach out: National programme student materials to support the delivery of training for psychological wellbeing practitioners delivering low intensity interventions. 3rd Edition.* Rethink Mental Illness.

Chapter 3

Being a Mental Health Wellbeing Practitioner

Introduction

This role-specific chapter introduces the newest of the psychological practitioner (PP) roles, the Mental Health Wellbeing Practitioner (MHWP). This is the most recent to be established and, like the Psychological Wellbeing Practitioner (PWP), is a practitioner role working with adults.

This chapter will focus on the strategies the MHWP can apply and in which settings. This includes clinical skills to assess and engage, as well as training to deliver low-intensity (LI) interventions. It will also explore the key difference between the PWP and MHWP roles in the training of MHWPs to contribute to care planning.

Kirsten Brown, a qualified MHWP, tells us

> The MHWP role is something exciting to be a part of, because it is in many ways groundbreaking. Being able to offer psychologically informed interventions to people to people who, in a surprisingly high number of cases, haven't been able to engage in talking therapies previously is a rewarding and empowering process for the service users, and for us as Practitioners.

The people Kirsten speaks of offering interventions to are adults with more severe mental health problems. When we say severe mental health, this can incorporate working with adults who have psychosis, bipolar disorder, or who are involved with drug and alcohol (D&A) services. We know that there is a significant unmet need for psychological interventions in this area of mental health,

DOI: 10.4324/9781003542049-3

and the MHWP role is designed to support this. It is based upon the PWP LI cognitive behavioural therapy (CBT)-informed model (which you can read about in Chapter 2); however, MHWPs are trained to deliver their interventions in the context of severe mental health.

Matthew Beaton, a Principal Mental Health Practitioner and Honorary Lecturer on an MHWP programme, tells us,

> This is a role that provides psychological interventions within Community Mental Health Teams (CMHTs), increasing access for individuals with more complex mental health needs and improving their quality of life. However, it also offers diverse professional experiences for practitioners, due to the variety of services that MHWPs work in, including but not limited to, CMHTs, crisis services, and D&A services.

Kirsten notes that sometimes service users have been within mental health services for many years but have not had the opportunity to engage with talking therapies, or sometimes they have not been made aware of how LI talking therapies can help them.

Adam Hope, a qualified MHWP, tells us that his favourite thing about the MHWP role is the opportunity to make a positive difference in the lives of individuals who have traditionally been overlooked by mental health services and may have 'fallen between the gaps' in terms of psychologically informed mental health care until now.

In addition to offering evidence-based interventions, MHWPs are also able to coordinate and contribute to care planning for the service users they support. This is a key difference between the MHWP and PWP roles and the training received.

Background

CMHTs offer community-based mental health support and treatment for adults with a range of mental health conditions. This may include short-term support or crisis intervention, or longer-term care for those with more enduring or severe difficulties.

Figures suggest that, out of all adults accessing CMHTs, no more than 3% have accessed an evidence-based psychological therapy in the past 12 months (figures not including early intervention in psychosis teams). This identified need for increased access to psychological support has been highlighted within the community transformation agenda, a national commitment to overhauling and transforming CMHTs and the community-based offer. The community transformation agenda is an integral part of the National Health Service (NHS) Long-Term Plan. The psychological professions census and NHS Long-Term Workforce Plan also show and continue to evidence this workforce need.

This identified need and the plans for change led to the development of the MHWP role, as part of a wider range of initiatives developed to enable CMHTs to transform. The role of the MHWP was designed to support a shift in services from generic care coordination towards more psychologically informed, meaningful intervention-based care. They also work from a trauma-informed approach within their role. The new role needed to have synergy with, but distinct competencies from, established roles, and it needed to be well-governed. Basing the role on the well-established PWP role, with its evidence-based offer, focus on wellbeing, and strong emphasis on supervision, allowed for this, whilst enabling the MHWP role to be adapted for the different target population.

The first cohort of MHWP trainees began in March 2022. The training places are, in most cases, recruit-to-train positions, which means that new staff are brought into the workforce (rather than training being offered to develop existing staff). Therefore, with each cohort of trainees, the overall community mental health workforce has also increased.

Adam Hope, a qualified MHWP, tells us about the benefits he sees in the role and how it can support a wider CMHT. He says,

> MHWPs offer low-intensity interventions to individuals with complex needs or vulnerabilities, therefore these individuals can now be seen relatively quickly or can be offered treatment prior to being seen by CBT therapists or Clinical Psychologists. This keeps waiting times down and helps to make the workload of senior practitioners more manageable and benefits the service user by making psychologically informed support accessible at a time when they really need it.

Scope and Remit

MHWPs are based in existing NHS teams and commissioned services. This includes the transformed CMHTs, as well as D&A services, perinatal teams, and eating disorder teams (although this is not an exhaustive list and may expand as this relatively new role develops and becomes more established).

MHWPs tend to be placed in smaller numbers in services, working alongside other professionals from a variety of roles. MHWPs are not placed in specific services, as PWPs are in NHS Talking Therapies (NHSTT, formerly Improving Access to Psychological Therapies or IAPT) or Educational Mental Health Practitioners (EMHPs) are in Mental Health Support Teams. The MHWP role therefore includes a considerable element of multidisciplinary team (MDT) working. MDT working can also be a function of other practitioner roles, as is the ability to work well within teams; however, it is referenced in most detail within this chapter due to its significance to the MHWP role.

MDTs can be found in many parts of the NHS; however, they are more commonly associated with secondary or tertiary care. An MDT is characterised by being made up of a group of professionals, from different disciplines, for example, psychological professionals, medics, nursing, social work, or allied health professionals, from both health and social care. They meet at regularly scheduled timepoints, working together to contribute and make decisions about the treatment of the service users in their care.

MHWPs are most often based within the transformed CMHTs, but whether based here or in other secondary care services (i.e., D&A), the role of MHWPs is to support adults of all ages who present with severe mental health problems (the definition of this having been discussed earlier).

The aim is that LI, PP support will help people towards recovery and to experience improvement in their lives. MHWPs work within their teams with service users, but also staff, to promote good mental health and recovery from severe mental health problems and to increase psychological understanding.

It is within the scope and remit of the MHWP to perform initial assessments and deliver one-to-one and group-based psychological interventions. MHWPs can offer evidence-based interventions, such as behavioural activation (BA), graded exposure (GE), and more.

MHWPs can also contribute to, support, collaborative care planning for the individuals they are working with.

During training, MHWPs are supported to develop skills which they can then use in care planning and coordination as part of the MDT within their services. This element of working is distinct and new for the MHWP role and is a key way in which the role provides improved access to psychologically informed support.

Alongside all the work that they do, MHWPs use Patient-Reported Outcome Measures (PROMs) to help assess and monitor progress and impact on service users. This is in keeping with routine outcome measures or the minimum data set embedded into the Children's Wellbeing Practitioner (CWP) and EMHP roles, PWP role, and the wider NHSTT and Children and Young People's Psychological Training (CYP PT, formerly Children and Young People's IAPT) programmes.

The main PROMs recommended for MHWP use are as follows:

- Recovering Quality of Life (ReQoL) for Users of Mental Health Services is a measure that gives a voice to the service user and makes them central to their recovery journey. It also provides the MHWP with a valid and reliable aid to clinical decision-making and outcome monitoring, with use recommended every session.
- Goal-based outcomes is used to ascertain whether the service user is getting where they want to with the interventions. It measures progress and outcome against the goal and is again recommended for use every session.
- DIALOG is a service-based measure (some services may use an alternative) to assess a service user's satisfaction in the life domains, for example, employment and relationships, that may be being impacted by their mental health. It also considers treatment aspects of the service users' care. As such, DIALOG provides a subjective measure of quality of life and treatment satisfaction.

MHWPs also require regular supervision from an appropriately qualified supervisor, which will be covered in more detail later in this chapter.

In addition to the interventions and care planning elements covered above, MHWPs may also be signposting to additional services, requiring good knowledge of the wider local offer available in their geographical area. As part of their role, they'll also work to incorporate families and carers in care plans or interventions, where this is appropriate to the service user.

It may be that adaptations are required to treatment to make it accessible to service users with severe or enduring mental health difficulties and additional complexities. MHWPs are trained and supported to do this whilst also ensuring that the interventions are still in line with the evidence base (this is known as ensuring fidelity to the model).

Common types of adaptations for MHWPs to consider might include adjusting language to make it more straightforward to understand, incorporating visual aids or worksheets to support elements of interventions, or slowing down the pace of the intervention and delivering it over additional sessions. MHWPs are encouraged to use supervision to consider adaptation and check fidelity to the evidence base.

Box 3.1   Adaptation in practice case example

One of our contributing MHWPs, who will remain unnamed to preserve the anonymity of the service user, tells us about an example of adaptation within practice:

"I worked with a young adult who had a learning disability (LD) as well as being registered blind. Some life experiences had left this person feeling low in mood and having quite poor self-esteem.

I was able to work with them across 12 sessions of low-intensity CBT (LI CBT), using creativity within the sessions to engage them and adapting the treatment to accommodate for this person's LD and their visual impairment.

I was closely supervised through this case and the adaptations made. I had some lovely feedback from my supervisor who told me they were very impressed, and that it was a great example of how LI CBT can benefit the service users we work with, in a way that is efficient and cost effective for the service".

MHWPs can provide their assessments and interventions through a variety of methods of delivery. These methods can include face-to-face delivery, either individually or in groups, via telephone, making use of an online platform for individual work, such as Attend Anywhere, Microsoft Teams, or Zoom, or via access to a computerised CBT platform. MHWPs in some areas are also currently involved in trials for making use of artificial intelligence video intervention to support treatment.

Population Served

The role and remit of an MHWP is to work specifically with adults, of any age and including older adults, who experience severe and enduring mental health conditions.

As the role has emerged and developed, there are now MHWPS working in a variety of more specialist secondary care services, including D&A, eating disorders, and learning disabilities. This still fits with the remit identified above, whilst acknowledging some of the more specific complexities that MHWPs in such a specialist service may encounter.

Adam Hope, a qualified MHWP, tells us about his work specifically within the support of people with learning disabilities. He says,

I love working with individuals with Learning Disabilities. Many of these service users have faced considerable adversity and have quite complex difficulties and co-morbidities. In the past they may have been considered a bad fit for psychological therapy. However, in my experience, these individuals have much to benefit from psychologically informed interventions and with some adaptation, these interventions can make a huge difference to people that are in real need of mental health support.

Specified System of Care

For MHWPs, the specified system of care in which they should work is a mental health service clearly identified as being for adults (this can include older adults) with severe mental health problems.

The two registering organisations for PP roles, the British Psychological Society (BPS) and the British Association of Behavioural and Cognitive Psychotherapies (BABCP), have recently launched registration for MHWPs, following in the footsteps of their sibling roles, PWP, CWP, and EMHP. Their guidance emphasises the need for MHWPs to work within this specified system of care, allowing for appropriate supervision and stepping of care where required. Guidance makes clear that MHWPs should not work in isolation.

Due to the more severe nature of mental health difficulties with which MHWP will be working, either in a care planning or intervention capacity, it is important that the systems in which they work give access for MHWPs to be able to immediately escalate concerns where they might arise. This could be in relation to concerns regarding a service user's (or others') safety (risk management). An alternative example could be concerns related to issues such as appropriately managing a medication review and prescribing, outside the remit of the MHWP, but where access to professionals within the MDT would be best placed to support the service user.

Supervision

MHWPs require regular supervision as part of their role, during their training period, and once qualified. Due to the MDT setting in which they work, there are a number of professionals who may be able to provide the different types of required supervision for MHWPs. A comprehensive list is available via the registering organisations (BPS and BABCP), but we have given a broad sense of the requirements within the descriptions of the types of supervision below. The two types of supervision are as follows.

Case Management Supervision (CMS)

This type of supervision is focused on reviewing the caseload of the MHWP, with an overview of the whole caseload and specific cases explored in more detail to allow appropriate next steps to be decided. CMS will give particular focus to the cases that the MHWP is involved in coordinating care for.

This supervision takes place weekly, for a minimum of one hour, and on an individual basis.

The case management supervisor can be any member of the MDT who is a qualified mental health professional and has training and experience of working with adults with severe mental health problems.

Psychological Intervention Supervision (PIS)

This type of supervision has a specific name, PIS, for MHWPs but is broadly similar to the clinical skills supervision undertaken by PWPs, CWPs, and EMHPs.

This type of supervision focuses on the development and maintenance of clinical skills specifically for cases where MHWPs are delivering CBT-informed psychological interventions. This is done through presentation and discussion of cases, role play of clinical interactions, and observation of others doing the same.

This type of supervision takes place fortnightly, for a minimum of one hour, and most often in groups. Where this supervision is held in groups, these should be no larger than six qualified MHWPs per group, and no more than three MHWPs per group for trainees.

The psychological intervention, or clinical skills, supervisor must be a psychological professional who is trained and experienced in the delivery of CBT-based interventions for severe mental health problems, who has also attended specific supervision training linked to the training programme. This may be the same person as the case management supervisor if they meet the criteria for both types of supervision.

Supervision hours may be amended pro rata for part-time MHWPs but should never be less than fortnightly in frequency, and supervision should never be less than 30 minutes per session (30 minutes of PIS and 30 minutes of CMS).

Adam Hope is a qualified MHWP and spoke to us about the benefits of supervision. He says, "Supervision allows you the space to reflect, to practice skills outside of the therapy room and provides a safe space to share your own thoughts about your practice which is essential for professional development". Adam notes how this was a change from his previous experience of supervision, saying

In my previous role as a support worker for individuals with autism and learning disabilities, supervision was limited to 6 monthly wellbeing check-ins, which were delivered over the phone. The supervision I have received as an MHWP has been much more frequent, focused, and structured. Supervision within this role is highly valued and is considered an important part of professional development. At times the role can be emotionally demanding, and supervision provides the opportunity to reflect on your own wellbeing and be supported with this.

Both during training and once qualified, it is expected that supervisors will see practitioners' live practice. This can be done via the supervisor joining a session, through watching a video recording, or through listening to an audio recording, and gives the supervisor an excellent opportunity to support the development of practice, as well as noting and giving feedback on practitioner strengths.

Pre-Intervention

Engagement and Assessment

MHWPs need to be able to respond to distress. Their training teaches them skills to recognise and explore the distress that their service users may present with. At this early stage in engagement, the MHWP is likely to be utilising their skills to validate the service users' experience, reflecting back and summarising to support shared understanding and the start of engagement building.

An MHWP will only begin further work when it is appropriate to proceed. The MHWP assessment is person-centred interviewing using the funnelling technique. This technique is based around using open questions at first before latterly moving to closed questions. Throughout the assessment interview process, MHWPs will summarise, clarify, use reflection, and provide feedback to the service user to ensure their shared understanding of the presenting difficulties and situation.

The MHWP is taught a range of models and approaches to support them in their engagement and assessment of service users.

The following will be discussed briefly below: 5Ps, Five Areas, Stress Bucket, CHIME, and Trauma-Informed Care (TIC).

A 5Ps formulation explores the services users presenting problem by considering the predisposing factors (factors that exist that contributed to its development), precipitating factors (that have come before), perpetuating factors (is keeping it going), and protective factors (that mitigate effect and harm).

MHWPs are also introduced to the 'Stress Bucket' metaphor to support their conversations about the 5Ps with service users. This metaphor sees the individual as a bucket made with their predisposing factors, with the water flowing into the bucket the precipitating factors. There are holes at the bottom of the bucket; those that are blocked represent perpetuating factors, and those that allow water to escape represent protective factors. If the water builds up and overflows, this indicates the presenting problem arising.

A five areas model is based on CBT principles. The model can be used to gather information about the service users' presentation in the key areas. It contains the four factors that make up the individual, so you have got your thoughts, feelings, physical symptoms, and behaviours. The model also includes the environmental factors, external to, but impacting on the individual. This can be a really insightful model to use with service users to help them see how these areas interact and impact upon each other. It helps to support the identification of perpetuating cycles that are part of the maintenance of the service users' symptoms. For example, an avoidance behaviour or a negative automatic thought, maintaining a feeling of low mood. It is also a useful model to help identify particular interventions that would help break a service user's vicious cycles and help build some virtuous cycles.

CHIME is an acronym, from research by Mary Leamy and colleagues, into understanding the factors considered important, by those with severe mental health problems, in contributing to their recovery. The five factors identified were as follows:

1 Connectedness
2 Hope and optimism about the future
3 Identity
4 Meaning (meaning in life and making sense of mental health issues)
5 Empowerment

The research also pointed to the importance of MHWPs considering these five factors within their person-centred interview with service users, alongside PROMs such as ReQoL, which also captures data on these factors.

As already referenced above, MHWPs work with a TIC approach. This approach is about recognising what trauma is and how it affects us. In relation to the service user, it involves recognising traumatic events they have experienced and the impact of these and responding appropriately without re-traumatising.

Problem Statement and Identifying Goals

At the end of the information gathering section of the person-centred interview, there is a shift to shared decision-making. We have mentioned at various points throughout this chapter the importance of collaboration and shared decision-making between the MHWPs and the service user they are supporting, and this really begins at this point.

The problem statement will cover three things: the context, the problem, and its impact. It should be drawn collaboratively from the information gathering section of the interview and is used as a reference point throughout intervention work.

From the problem statement, the MHWP can start to consider what support the service user may benefit from and begin to consider this with them. It is important that the support and interventions meet and are adapted to the service user's problem statement and individual needs.

Risk Assessment

Risk assessment occurs throughout the service user's care journey. There is a need to risk assess to ensure the service user receives appropriate care and support, as risk can fluctuate and change over time. This could be a topic of several books in its own right, and therefore, this is only a very brief overview of the topic.

It is important not to be afraid of asking questions in terms of risk assessment; research shows that asking about suicide does not increase the risk of service users acting on these thoughts. There are ways in which MHWPs can approach this topic and build rapport with the service user, to ask the right questions at the right time, making them supportive, meaningful, and protective for the service user. Once this information is gathered, an MHWP, with the support of supervision and the MDT, can work to consider the best treatment options for the service user and can work with the service user to create a risk management plan (this will form part of their care plan – see below). The MHWP must take a collaborative approach to identifying and managing risks. This can include opportunities for the service user to take positive risks and self-manage, with plans to support the mitigation of risk, whilst also an awareness of how any immediate risk should be managed.

In April 2025, NHS England published 'Staying safe from suicide'; this guidance co-produced with service user and public voice promotes a person-centred approach with a focus on understanding a person's situation and managing safety.

It is important for MHWPs to also understand, be informed, and be able to act in accordance with Safeguarding Adults and Safeguarding Children policies and procedures.

Care Planning

Contributing to care planning is part of the MHWP role. As with other aspects of the MHWP role, this should be a collaborative process with the service user, alongside other members of the MDT. It is also worth noting here the importance of the sharing of information, with the right people, at the right time; this could be, but not limited to, other family members, carers, health and care professionals.

The care plan is the written record reflecting the outcome of the assessment, identified needs, and goals, as discussed above. It should also cover the options explored and the plans or actions to be taken. It is important that the care plan is regularly, formally, and informally reviewed; it is a living document and should reflect the service user's current needs.

Triangle of Care, Considering the Role of the Carer

In the settings in which MHWPs work, the service users are likely to have family and friends, or others, providing various forms and levels of support and or care. Working with family and or carer involvement, in a family-inclusive approach, is therefore an important part of the MHWPs remit.

The Triangle of Care model, introduced to NHS services in 2023, highlights the need for carer support and inclusion in secondary care mental health services. The Triangle of Care focuses on unpaid carers, but many of the principles would apply to paid carers. Furthermore, it demonstrates that excluding carers can have a negative impact, leading to missing information and reduced intervention effectiveness. Conversely, involving carers can support therapeutic engagement and improvements in intervention effectiveness and outcomes.

In a case example provided by a practicing MHWP, fully anonymised and using a pseudonym, Sienna, which is not the service user's real name, and Matilda, her carer, demonstrated how Matilda's involvement helps to mitigate risk. By ensuring that Matilda was informed and aligned with the therapeutic goals and strategies, it supported the management of Sienna's vulnerabilities and, in this case, helped to prevent potential exploitation or abuse. Actively involving Matilda in the care plan allowed the MDT to benefit from her support. Excluding Matilda may have meant missing out on critical information that could enhance Sienna's therapy and overall wellbeing. The MHWP reflected on Sienna's case that by applying principles of the Triangle of Care model, the MHWP recognised the critical role of Matilda in Sienna's emotional and psychological support.

Signposting

Signposting can play an important part of the MHWP role. As practitioners deliver LI interventions, it is not possible or appropriate to do everything!

So what is signposting and how can it be done well in practice?

Signposting can be utilised through both the assessment and treatment process, for example, to community organisations or peer support. It may also be used where a service user may benefit from support and direction to engage with a recovery college or educational opportunity. Signposting should always be tailored to the needs of the individual, and there are far too many options to list here, and these will vary between areas and regions.

That is why knowing your local area is key. It is also important to have an understanding of the quality and relevance of services you may signpost to, and some questions you could ask yourself are as follows:

Who are your service users?

What are their specific needs?

What is available in your area?

Are the services able and appropriately qualified to offer the services they advertise?

Is it free or low cost?

Finally, how do you and your service update and review knowledge of local services, particularly as there are often funding changes, other financial pressures, criteria changes, or, waiting list closures that impact on the delivery of services in the community?

Interventions

Below are some summaries and examples of the interventions MHWPs use within their practice. Though the choice and frequency of use may be influenced by the setting the MHWP is working in, as well as, of course, the individual they are working with, intervention mapping and shaping should be done using a shared decision-making approach with the service user.

BA Using the "GOALS" Programme

BA is an evidence-based treatment for low mood and depression that is used across the PP roles, including MHWP. There is a strong evidence base supporting the effectiveness of BA, either as a stand-alone intervention (as an MHWP might deliver) or as a component of a high-intensity CBT intervention.

Box 3.2   BA case example from practice

An example of a low-mood case from practice has been provided by a practicing MHWP, who will remain unnamed to preserve the anonymity of the service user they supported. The case example below is fully anonymised and makes use of a pseudonym, John, which is not the service user's real name.

> "John, a middle-aged, white, male, was under the care of the CMHT with longstanding difficulties with his mental health and multiple admissions for inpatient care in his history (many years previously). John had been offered, and accessed, counselling and psychotherapy previously, more than once, but reported not finding any benefit to this.
>
> John agreed to meet with an MHWP for assessment, with the presenting problem identified as low mood. John had previously experienced some anxiety following the lockdowns associated with the 2020 pandemic, and since that time had found himself limited in activity. Things that John had previously enjoyed, including swimming, days out, and family holidays, were things he was no longer doing.
>
> John was able to tell his MHWP that he would have thoughts around not being able to do things or go to places that he didn't know. He shared that he would often think that there was no hope of getting back to his former self. This caused John to feel sad, hopeless, disengaged, and stuck. John described how he would withdraw and spend less time out of the house and would avoid doing the things he used to enjoy".

BA aims to target avoidance and re-establish routine in service users experiencing symptoms of low mood or depression.

In depression, a vicious cycle is created; it is reinforced through avoidance of activity and reduced opportunity for positive reinforcement. BA helps break that cycle and create a more virtuous one.

1 Understand how depression impacts personal goals.
2 Set personal goals for BA – what does the service user want to do more of?
3 Break down goals – make sure you are using SMART principles (Chapter 11).
4 Complete steps.
5 Review progress.

GE Using the "GOALS" Programme

GE is an intervention that can be offered by MHWPs for anxiety presentations where avoidance is a key factor in keeping the problem going (maintenance of the problem). The avoidance of situations and or objects due to fear only provides short-term relief from the anxiety symptoms, and longer term is a maintaining factor. GE is the planned therapeutic confrontation of a feared situation or object. The GE intervention is based on supporting the service user to have gradually increasing amounts of contact with the object or situation causing anxiety.

The GOALS programme approach is highlighted in the five steps below:

1   Understand how anxiety impacts the personal goals of the service user.
2   Set personal goals for the GE: what avoidance does the service user want to overcome?
3   Build an anxiety ladder or hierarchy, with the steps building towards the goal.
4   Service user works to complete the steps.
5   Review progress.

There are three factors that should be considered for the successful implementation of the GE intervention:

Prolonged – enough time for the anxiety symptoms to reduce (at least a 50% reduction) in the presence of a situation or an object.

Repeated – it is not enough to do the task once.

Without distraction – the individual must experience a level of fear to be able to notice the reduction.

The MHWP begins by supporting the service user to plan actions to achieve steps on their hierarchy in the session. The MHWP should be mindful that goals and steps should be appropriately paced, and potentially broken down into smaller steps, to ensure that the service user does not trigger high levels of anxiety, as this can be associated with relapse of severe mental health problems. Then starting with the least anxiety provoking step, the MHWP supports the service user to begin the GE tasks. This may initially be with the service user, without becoming part of the avoidance, moving to between-session activities, with the service user remaining in the situation until they experience habituation.

Below is a case study that utilises the GE intervention. It also highlights the processes that the MHWP took to come to the shared decision with the service user to undertake GE:

Box 3.3   Graded exposure case example from practice

This case study has been provided by a practicing MHWP, who will remain unnamed to preserve the anonymity of the service user they supported. The case example below is fully anonymised.

Female, 30 years, living with partner. Long-term anxiety relating to severe mental health condition. Came in for sessions due to increased anxiety after receiving two speeding fines in short succession. The incidents happened during journeys to work.

Thoughts:

"I am going to get into trouble from the Police if I drive my car"
    "There are too many cameras and Police cars about"
    "I can't risk not having my licence"

Feelings/Physical Sensations:

Heart rate increased, sweaty, shaky, chest pains
    Panic, worry, fear, dread

Behaviours:

Avoid driving to work – ask my partner or a colleague to give me a lift
    When I do drive, I am tense and looking out for speed cameras and police cars (hypervigilance)

Walk to places or use public transport rather than drive to reduce the chance of something bad happening whilst driving

Impact:

Feeling out of control
   Reduction in independence
   Impact on relationships – I feel I am burdening my partner and colleagues
   Feeling I am wasting money on my car and increased spending on public transport
   Not wanting to go out as much as I used to as it feels much more difficult now than it used to

Chosen intervention:

Psychoeducation *around the fight-flight response and avoidance cycle*
   Five areas formulation *– understanding relationships between thoughts, feelings, body sensations, and behaviours*

Graded Exposure:

Firstly creating an understanding of the goal(s) the service user had and an introduction to what habituation is (understanding how slow and steady exposure can help to reduce anxiety).

Identifying anxiety-provoking situations and making a hierarchy of them – most to least feared.

Understanding what safety behaviours are in place and why they are in place. Also, exploring how although they may be helpful to manage anxiety, they may not allow us to truly face the anxiety provoking to habituate to it.

Planning the exposure – breaking this down into manageable chunks, considering exposure being prolonged, repeated, and without distraction. Asking the service user to complete an exposure diary for homework. Rating the anxiety before the anxiety-provoking situation, during, and after.

*Reviewing the exposure diary and considering barriers that may have gotten in the way of completing exposure? Was this approach helpful? Does this feel like something that we can keep adding to? – Using a **problem-solving** approach here.*

Introducing grounding techniques here to support the service user to manage physical experiences of anxiety to support the service user to be more likely to exposure self to anxiety-provoking situations.

Review goals set and consider progress – focusing on the wins the service user has had (even if the service user perceives them to be small).

Outcomes:

The service user reported that using the five areas formulation to consider the relationships between thoughts, feelings, body sensations, and behaviours was helpful. This helped to make sense of why driving was a difficulty for the service user, based on all of the four areas and not just based off the anxious thoughts the service user was experiencing.

The use of Graded Exposure across our eight sessions allowed us to approach the goal(s) at an appropriate pace for the service user. Allowing for us to have chance to explore possible barriers that may have been getting in the way and consider ways of problem-solving these too.

Teaching Problem-Solving Skills

As seen in the case study above, problem-solving is a practical approach that MHWPs can teach to service users. It can be particularly useful if there are practical or situational factors impacting on the service user's mental health.

The role of MHWPs is not to solve the service users' problem(s) for them but to teach them the seven-step problem-solving approach, as a strategy, to allow the service user to gain the skill in their toolkit to solve their problems, particularly when problems are identified by the service user as being too big to solve, initially.

The problem-solving approach works through a seven-step process, and it can be beneficial to encourage the service user to write down notes to help them work through the steps in a systematic way and to help them gain some additional clarity that may be more challenging if they are anxious, low, or worrying, and this is impacting on their thought processes.

The steps are outlined below:

1 Identify the problem
2 Identify the solution
3 Analyse strengths and weaknesses
4 Select a solution
5 Plan implementation
6 Implementation
7 Review

It may initially appear straightforward, especially if you yourself are not feeling low or anxious, but it can be a powerful intervention to add to someone's toolkit in practice.

Encouraging Sleep

Good quality sleep is a key foundation to mental and physical wellbeing; conversely, poor sleep can be the result of, or contribute to, poor physical and mental wellbeing. When completing an assessment with a service user, questions around sleep will be part of the assessment. MHWPs can also utilise the Insomnia Severity Index. It is important to consider both the amount and quality of the sleep a service user is getting. Diaries may help not only to establish patterns and trigger but also to monitor progress with the intervention.

For MHWPs, there are three factors that are key to encouraging good sleep:

1 Timing
2 Sleep pressure
3 Feeling relaxed and calm

The stages for MHWPs to then use to support a service user to improve their sleep can be broken into key areas: identifying factors that disrupt, setting the sleep window, building sleep pressure, and feeling calm and relaxed. As the intervention progresses, it is important to review progress.

Difficulties with sleep are often a factor in both anxiety and depression presentations. Changes and improvements to achieve more restful and effective sleep can be beneficial both to mood symptoms and enable service users to feel more resourced to engage in interventions; therefore, it can be a good foundation to complete with a service user or an intervention for sleep as a main problem in its own right.

Recognising and Managing Emotions

We all experience emotions, feeling a whole range: happy, sad, angry ..., and the list could go on. When we experience an emotion that is in keeping with the experience and intensity for the situation, we call this regulated. When our emotion is out of sync with our experience, is too intense or absence, or is associated with a previous experience, we call this dysregulated, for example, feeling upset when something has gone well. Emotional dysregulation can feel overwhelming.

MHWPs can work with the service user, at their invitation, on developing skills in emotional regulation. This is where the emotional response can be increased or decreased when the individual wants it to be. The intervention is not about telling the service user how to feel. It focuses on the emotion that the service user wants to and considers that emotion in relation to its usefulness in terms of the level at which it is being experienced.

In order to do this, MHWPs can support the service user to first recognise their emotions through the following means, helping and teaching the service user to:

1 Name emotions
2 Understand the function of each emotion
3 Check whether the emotion itself is appropriate to the situation
4 Check if the level of intensity is appropriate to the situation
5 How to increase or decrease the intensity of the emotion

Secondly, MHWPs are then taught to use a range of skills to support service users develop their emotional regulation, including opposite action and problem-solving (discussed above).

A composite example of this from practice is a service user who has experienced abuse, struggling with emotional reactions and regulation due to the impact of previous experience on the here and now. By supporting the individual to understand their emotions with more clarity and teaching them skills to manage them, they improved their emotional stability. In this example, this initial work served as a platform to build on to facilitate further positive change.

Building Confidence

Confidence can be defined as a self-assurance and appreciation of one's own abilities and qualities. It requires us to hold positive beliefs about ourselves, that is, that we are likable, have purpose. If we experienced difficulties in our lives, for example, the impact of a service user's mental health on their ability to engage with activity, more negative beliefs and views can begin to become more prevalent. There is evidence that these negative self-beliefs can be counter-balanced by more positive self-beliefs.

The MHWPs' 'Building Confidence' intervention focuses on principles from positive psychology, bringing focus to awareness of our strengths, values, and positive experiences, and incorporating these into daily life.

It can be used where low confidence is identified by the service user as part of the assessment as a specific goal but also where confidence is a factor in maintaining symptoms, for example, low mood.

The intervention can be considered in the six steps outlined below:

1   Assessing psychological wellbeing, that is, using the ReQoL-10, which, in addition to measuring wellbeing more broadly, has a specific item on confidence that could be useful when implementing this intervention
2   Identifying the service users' values and strengths
3   Making an activities list: this involves considering how to bring the service users' values and strengths into day-to-day actions
4   Planning the use of these actions during the weeks. These could be smaller things intended to be done regularly or larger things less frequently

5   Pay attention to the positives. For example, the introduction of a positive data log to support the noticing of positives in the day to day
6   Review progress with the service user, incorporating measures such as ReQoL-10

Guided Self-Help for Bulimia and Binge Eating

Included in the early curriculum for MHWPs is the use of guided self-help for eating disorders (GSH-ED). This is based on CBT principles. The GSH-ED is for use with service users presenting with bulimia nervosa and binge eating disorder. It contains work on topics such as eating patterns and body image.

In speaking to MHWPs during the writing of this book, feedback was that this intervention is used less frequently, more likely in specialist services, and with close supervisory support.

Medication Support

Service users in secondary care are likely to be prescribed medication as part of their treatment plan and to have their own thoughts and feelings related to their prescribed pharmacological interventions; therefore, it is important for MHWPs to be aware of the pharmacological treatments for anxiety, depression, psychosis, and bipolar. As well as awareness, the role of MHWPs is that of basic information giving, to service users, family members, and carers, to support service users to gain the best therapeutic outcome.

It is very important to be very clear with service users about the boundaries and limitations of this advice. MHWPs are not medical professionals or prescribers; however, being able to gather information and open up helpful communication around, for example, perceived medication issues, and supporting the service user to seek further professional input from the MDT can be valuable to the service user's overall care.

Qualification, Agenda for Change, and Registration

There are currently significant challenges to traditional recruitment in secondary care in the NHS. As stated at the beginning of this chapter, the role of the MHWP aims to tap into a different, new pool of workforce with more locally sourced recruitment and also widening access to psychological professional roles for people who may have previously not been eligible for training, but have other value to bring, for example, lived and living experience.

Qualification

The MHWP qualification can be taken at a level 6 or 7, with BPS course accreditation, leading to an MHWP qualification at either GradCert or PGCert, depending on entry level.

More information on routes into the profession is covered in Chapter 6.

Adam Hope came from a psychology degree to complete his MHWP training but notes, "trainees without a graduate level education and those that have been outside of education for a while, worried they might find the academic work quite challenging, can access support available to help with academic writing skills etc.", reassuring for those considering beginning an MHWP career journey, with less academic experience.

As well as written academic components, the training includes Observed Structured Clinical Examination, role play of both a psychological assessment and a wellbeing-based intervention. Adam told us that he felt "very nervous when being evaluated in this way' however, the feedback he was given enabled him 'to improve each time and feel that the experience has made me a better practitioner".

Adam reflects that the best thing about the MHWP training course was

> meeting other trainee's all from varied backgrounds and working in a diverse range of services and hearing about their experiences. The course provides you with a good educational basis and general understanding of mental health that can be applied in many settings.

Agenda for Change

Agenda for Change (AfC) is the NHS pay system, which was introduced to standardise pay and conditions for NHS workers.

Those MHWPs within NHS services will be paid on AfC Bands. For trainees, this is AfC Band 4, and, once qualified, MHWPs are paid at AfC Band 5. MHWPs employed in other non-NHS organisations, for example, voluntary community and social enterprise commissioned providers of D&A services, may have slightly different pay and conditions of employment.

Registration

MHWP registration became mandated in June 2025. As with the other PP roles, MHWPs have a choice of a professional body with whom they can register. Registration is available with either the BPS or the BABCP.

In order to register, MHWPs need to have completed a BPS-accredited MHWP course, be working with the specified system of care, and be receiving the specified type and frequency of supervision. At the point of re-registration, MHWPs need to demonstrate that over the previous 12 months they have completed the required amount of appropriate continuing professional development activity.

More information on the specifics of registration is covered in Chapter 9, Professional Ethics, and in Chapter 11, Starting Out.

Conclusion

We hope that this chapter has given you a good insight into the MHWP role and what this can look like in practice. Is this the PP role for you?

If not, please revisit Chapter 2 to consider the other adult practitioner role, the PWP, or continue on to Chapters 4 and 5 to explore the children and young people's practitioner roles, the CWP and EMHP.

If the MHWP role does sound like a good fit, then that's wonderful and welcome to the MHWP family – you may want to move on to Chapter 6 and beyond to continue exploring your career options.

Box 3.4   References and wider reading

Leamy, M., Bird, V., Le Boutillier, C., Williams, J., & Slade, M. (2011). Conceptual framework for personal recovery in mental health: Systematic review and narrative synthesis. *British Journal of Psychiatry*, 199 (6), pp. 445–452.

NHS England. (2022). *Mental health and wellbeing practitioner: A guide to practice*. NHS England. https://www.hee.nhs.uk/sites/default/files/documents/Mental%20Health%20and%20Wellbeing%20%20Practitioner%20A%20Guide%20to%20Practice.pdf

NHS England. (2023). *NHS long term workforce plan*. NHS England.

NHS England. (2023). *National curriculum for mental health and wellbeing practitioners*. NHS England.

NHS England. (2025). *Psychological professions national workforce census*. NHS England. https://www.england.nhs.uk/publication/psychological-professions-workforce-census/

Chapter 4

Being a Children's Wellbeing Practitioner

Introduction and Background

In 2017, Health Education England commissioned training for a new post, the children's wellbeing practitioner (CWP). The aim of the CWP role was to create a new cohort of psychological practitioners (PPs) who could provide low-intensity (LI) cognitive behavioural therapy (CBT)-informed interventions to children and young people (YP) who were experiencing mild to moderate common mental health difficulties.

This role not only drew on the experiences and early indications of success in the adult Improving Access to Psychological Therapies (IAPT) programme and psychological wellbeing practitioner (PWP) role but also aimed to replicate some of the elements of the model, such as the presenting problems being targeted (anxiety and depression primarily) and the brief duration of support given.

The expansion to include training for the CWP role developed the Children and Young People's IAPT (CYP IAPT) offer further. CYP IAPT was established in 2011 alongside the publication 'No Health Without Mental Health'. 'No Health Without Mental Health' set out the government's aims and objectives for improving mental health and wellbeing outcomes, and services, with an emphasis on early intervention, prevention, and making use of organisations outside of the NHS (sometimes referred to as third sector organisations) to put this into place.

DOI: 10.4324/9781003542049-4

Box 4.1 Quote

By promoting good mental health and intervening early, particularly in the crucial childhood and teenage years, we can help to prevent mental illness from developing and mitigate its effects when it does.

No Health Without Mental Health:
A cross-government strategy (2011)

By 2017, CYP IAPT was training psychological therapists in CBT, parenting training, systemic family practice, and interpersonal psychotherapy for adolescents. These ranges of therapies are often referred to as high-intensity (HI).

The CYP IAPT programme had been rolled out into existing Child and Adolescent Mental Health Services (CAMHS) teams, as a service transformation programme. This meant that staff were being trained from within existing staff teams, developing their skills and competencies (be that in an HI psychological therapy, supervision, or leadership), and enhancing the evidence-based offer from the service. This was different from the adult IAPT programme, where new services were developed at Step 2 to 'house' the newly trained staff and develop a new and distinct offer.

The addition of the CWP role provided the programme with a new LI strand. As with the HI therapists being trained, CWPs were included in the service transformation model and added to existing teams.

The development of the CWP role was also aligned with the aims of The Five Year Forward View (2014) and the subsequent Mental Health Taskforce report (2016), which outlined the need for a significant expansion of the workforce in Children and Young People's Mental Health (CYPMH), in order to close the gap between what was needed (demand) and what evidence-based support was available (provision). Reports at this time were indicating how specialist CAMHS were struggling to meet the increasing demands for help and the increase in complexity in cases, meaning that waiting lists to see mental health professionals were growing significantly.

The NHS England and Department of Health report Future in Mind, published in 2015, gave recommendations on what needed to be done to improve the ways in which children's mental health and wellbeing could be supported. The report stated that, when ill, children and YP should receive good quality and timely care.

Launching CWP and expanding the workforce with PPs trained in offering evidence-based support, as early intervention, and for a brief duration, was one of the methods of achieving this increase in access to timely, effective care.

Lettie Smyth, a qualified CWP and supervisor, shares her thoughts on the value of the CWP role and early intervention. She tells us, "I believe prevention is key to supporting wellbeing, and the introduction of early intervention work is not only helping young people but also helping to educate the adults around those young people that we see".

Lettie goes on to say the role allows her to offer skills and knowledge that can be built upon in adulthood, perhaps creating a more stable foundation for a YP to succeed from. She adds,

> The idea of supporting children and young people also feels like a step in the right direction regarding battling stigma and normalising the idea of seeking advice. Surely generational exposure to the idea of seeking help can only break down negative beliefs about accessing therapy.

CWP courses have been training since 2017. Training places are, in most cases, recruit-to-train positions, which means that new staff are brought into the workforce (rather than training being offered to develop existing staff). Therefore, with each cohort of trainees, the overall CYPMHS workforce also increases.

This service transformation is all underpinned by a set of principles for working, initially referred to as the CYP IAPT Principles, updated recently to Children and Young People's Psychological

Training Principles, with the move away from the term IAPT. The principles are as follows:

- **Accessibility**
  This involves increasing the amount of access for YP and families to mental health and wellbeing support.
- **Accountability**
  This encourages the use of outcome measurement (via routine outcome measures or ROMs) to hold services accountable for their work.
- **Awareness**
  This emphasises the need to increase awareness of mental health issues and tackle stigma around mental ill-health in children and YP.
- **Evidence-Based Practice**
  This is a commitment to providing support and interventions that have a strong evidence base and keeping up to date with developments and changes in evidence.
- **Participation**
  This supports valuing and facilitating the active involvement of children, YP, parents, carers, and communities, at both an individual and a service level.

These principles are designed to work together, rather than independently, to ensure that they support and enhance the overall culture of CYPMH services.

An additional crucial aspect of the CWP role (and indeed all PP roles) is to ensure that all YP, parents, carers, and families are treated with respect and dignity, irrespective of any actual or perceived difference in characteristic, status, or element of their identity. This is often captured within cultural competency or responsiveness, or equality, diversity, and inclusion, and is also incorporated into the codes of conduct and ethical practice for both registering bodies for PPs, the British Psychological Society and the British Association of Behavioural and Cognitive Psychotherapies.

Safa Asif is a qualified CWP and tells us that her own identity, as a Muslim from a South Asian background, with lived experience of mental health issues within her family, was part of the reason she wanted to train in the role. Safa explains

> There are not many people of colour within the mental health field, which is much needed as those from ethnic diverse communities are at higher risk of developing mental health issues. There is a massive stigma within different cultures and communities, and I wanted to make sure I could tap into this and create that awareness and understanding. They are often labelled as 'hard to reach' but in fact, we are hard to reach. I wanted to change this, bringing in my own experiences and culture, to help adapt my work with the young people.

Scope and Remit

The remit of a CWP is to work with children and YP experiencing mild to moderate common mental health difficulties, including anxiety, low mood, and behavioural difficulties. CWPs can work directly with YP (where this is appropriately supported by the evidence base) or offer work with the parent or carer.

CWPs are trained to comprehensively assess risk in all cases at the first point of contact and to check in on risk at each subsequent contact. However, it should be emphasised that the role is neither appropriate nor designed for the ongoing support of YP presenting with current risk to themselves or others, or significant levels of historic risk.

The role is also not designed to support YP with serious or enduring mental health problems, or those requiring a more specialist level of care. CWPs can offer early intervention, for those with a first incidence of, or recently presenting, mild to moderate common mental health difficulties, where a brief intervention is likely to make a difference.

What does brief intervention mean? The guidance suggests that CWPs will generally offer somewhere in the region of six to eight sessions, with an assessment included within this. However, it may be that slightly fewer (four or less) or slightly more (up to ten) sessions are appropriate, with the nature of CWP interventions being described as focused but flexible.

Within their role, CWPs have the scope to work directly in person, face to face with YP, and families, in a range of community settings (such as youth centres, health centres, community venues, etc.) close to where these families live. This ties in with improving accessibility to evidence-based psychological treatment, and the key underpinning principles of the service transformation programme and the CWP role.

CWPs are also trained to offer support via remote methods, including telephone or online platforms such as MS Teams, Zoom, or service-specific secure platforms. These remote methods can supplement face-to-face work or can be utilised for a full intervention where this makes accessing the support more possible than it may be otherwise.

CWPs are trained to offer individual support, working one to one with YP, or parents and carers. The key CWP interventions of behavioural activation (BA), worry management (WM), and exposure (more details on these further on in this chapter) are all suitable for one-to-one support.

However, it is crucial to note here that even where intervention is primarily offered one to one directly with a YP, we know that YPs have parents, carers, and support systems around them that must also be considered. This means that CWPs, even when offering an individual intervention, will often include parents, carers, or other appropriate adults, in their sessions, or link these key adults with the sessions via additional face-to-face contact or phone calls. Evidence suggests that this involvement of key adults to support work outside of the weekly sessions can enhance the likelihood of improved outcomes.

CWPs can also offer group-based support, with this being included in the training curriculum since it was developed into a diploma in 2023 (see Chapter 8 – Being a Trainee for further details). Group support may involve delivery to YP or to parents and carers.

As well as offering these different types of direct intervention, the remit of a CWP includes a significant element of assessment, followed up by signposting to other types of support. This will be discussed in more detail further in this chapter.

An element of support that is specific to the CWP role is the community engagement and community-based work. This involves CWPs working outside of traditional clinic settings, to engage with local communities and support the mental health and wellbeing of YP in accessible, community-based venues.

More detail is given on this aspect of CWP work further on in this chapter.

Population Served

CWPs are trained to work with YP up to the age of 18 years, as well as with their parents or carers directly.

Individual interventions may target specific age ranges in line with the supporting evidence base. For example, the Brief Behavioural Activation (Brief BA) manualised intervention (Pass & Reynolds, 2021) that is often taught on CWP programmes is targeted specifically at adolescents.

There are also specific age ranges identified for the taught parent-led interventions, where the evidence base supports working with parents instead of the child, generally up to the age of 10 or 12 years.

Specified Systems of Care and Supervision

In the early years of CWP training (circa 2017 to around 2022), trainees were employed by NHS services and placed within or alongside CAMHS teams as part of the service transformation programme. There were some examples of trainees being placed in CAMHS partnership organisations, such as charities or community-based settings also.

In the last two years, there has been a focus on developing the CWP role into that of a community specialist practitioner, offering support to YP outside of traditional clinical settings and instead working via community organisations or primary care settings. There is more detail about this aspect of the role further on in this chapter.

In relation to the THRIVE Framework, a model for CYPMHS that has been rolled out across the past decade alongside wider service transformation work, the CWP role aligns most clearly to the 'Getting Advice' and 'Getting Help' quadrants. However, the role also supports the remaining areas of the model, 'Thriving', 'Getting More Help', and 'Getting Risk Support'. Further sources for reading on the Thrive model are included at the end of this chapter.

Where CWPs are employed by NHS Trusts, they are paid at NHS Agenda for Change pay band 4 during their training year, rising to pay band 5 for qualified CWPs. Salary in non-NHS organisations is generally broadly aligned to these rates of pay but may vary slightly.

It is important to note that a requirement of the CWP role is that practitioners work within systems of care that provide appropriate pathways to further care where needed. This is often referred to as stepped care and ensures that CWPs are not left holding cases that are outside the remit of their role, such as those with more severe mental health difficulties needing more intensive psychological therapy or a wider package of care. This model of stepped care is in fitting with the design of the PWP role (see Chapter 2 for further details).

A further specification of the systems in which CWPs work is that there is appropriate clinical governance (which broadly means ways of checking practice and ensuring best outcomes for YP and families) and that accountability for professional practice is held by a senior member of staff. Compared to PP roles that are embedded into a specific service structure, such as PWPs in Step 2 services (see Chapter 2 for further details) or EMHPs in Mental Health Support Teams (see Chapter 5 for further details), CWPs tend to be based in a wider variety of services which can mean that the senior members of staff have a more varied range of backgrounds. They may be HI cognitive behavioural therapists, CAMHS Practitioners with core backgrounds in nursing, social work, or occupational therapy, or clinical psychologists.

However, we are now also reaching the stage in the lifespan of the CWP role that qualified CWPs are staying with the role and going on to train as supervisors and senior wellbeing practitioners (SWPs – see Chapter 12 for further details). So, in more cases, now the senior member of staff directly supervising and overseeing CWP work may also have a background and training in LI CBT and the CWP role themselves.

Clinical supervision is offered frequently for CWPs and is distinct from line management supervision (LMS). Where LMS can generally be provided by anyone in a management position, clinical supervision must be provided by an appropriately qualified, experienced practitioner who usually also has training in CBT-informed practice.

Clinical supervision takes two forms:

- Clinical Case Management Supervision
  This is focused on reviewing the caseload of the CWP. For qualified CWPs, this should be offered at a minimum of one hour per fortnight and should be delivered individually.
- Clinical Skills Supervision
  This is focused on developing the skills of the CWP. It is generally provided in a group format, with no more than four CWPs in the group and a minimum of 30 minutes per practitioner. It should be offered at a minimum of one hour per fortnight for the first six months post-qualification and thereafter a minimum of one hour per month.

Another key specification is that referral pathways to CWPs should be distinct from existing referral routes to specialist CAMHS services, due to the differing criteria for CWP-appropriate cases. This ensures that cases being picked up by CWPs for assessment are most likely to be suitable to receive a brief, LI CBT-informed intervention, in line with the evidence base. Referrals received by CWPs should be presenting with a primary problem of anxiety or low mood, with a recent onset of the problem, and minimal to no risk present.

The CWP National Implementation Guide notes that emphasis on early intervention is key, and the CWP role should not include taking on work with more complex and severe mental health conditions. It continues to say that these more complex and severe presentations should be addressed in specialist CAMHS (or CYPMH services).

Pre-Intervention

Assessment

CWP assessments are based upon a CBT model, with a focus on the here and now of the presenting problem and identification of the factors that are keeping it going (also called maintenance factors). Although it can be beneficial to develop an understanding of the longer-term background of the YP who is seeking help (sometimes called a developmental history), this is not the primary goal of a CWP assessment.

CBT is fundamentally based upon the principle that the thoughts an individual has will impact on how they feel, both emotionally and physically, and this will, in turn, impact upon the things that they do (their behaviours). It is therefore key to a CBT-informed assessment to try and identify the thoughts, feelings (emotions and physical feelings in the body), and behaviours that occur in relation to the problem at hand.

One method of identifying the thoughts, feelings, and behaviours can be to ask the YP to think of the most recent time they have experienced the presenting problem. Using a specific example can help the YP to more clearly recall what thoughts and feelings they may have had, and what they did as a result. Keeping it recent makes this easier to do. This is sometimes referred to as completing a problem analysis or a recent incident analysis (RIA).

You may use questioning techniques such as funnelling, where a broad open question is asked first and then you 'funnel' down to further detail by using more specific and closed questions. You may use Socratic questioning, which helps to guide a YP or parent to make their own links and develop their own understanding of the problem and is known to be very effective. Questioning techniques such as the 'W questions' (what, where, when, with whom, etc.) or FIDO (asking about frequency, intensity, duration, and onset of the problem) can also be utilised in gathering information.

When going into assessment with a YP or parent/carer, you should always include an overview of confidentiality and the ways in which information about the YP will be recorded and stored. Best practice is to check with YPs what, if any, understanding they have of the word 'confidentiality' first, before then clarifying what it means and when information may not be able to be kept confidential (often referred to as 'breaking confidentiality'). It is important to do this at the start of the appointment, so that YP or parent/carers are aware of what might happen before they begin to share things with you.

As well as gathering information on the presenting problem, an initial assessment is a good opportunity for you to start to engage with the YP and build rapport. Asking about hobbies and interests, friendships, experience of school, and extra-curricular activities can give insight into the YP's life. Understanding who the YP has around them, in their family, living at home, and as a system of support, can also be part of this. You may use an activity such as creating a genogram, or family tree, to capture this information. This may also be an appropriate time to understand any difficult relationships the YP might have in their life. If parents are present in an assessment, they may also be able to provide an understanding of any mental health difficulties in the family. This can be helpful as we know from research that some presenting difficulties may be more likely to occur where there are similar difficulties in other members of the family, as well as some behavioural elements of problems being reinforced (kept going) by others, or potentially learned vicariously (which means from others).

Risk assessment is an important part of a CWP initial assessment, ensuring that risk is appropriately assessed and managed the first time you have contact with a child, YP, or family. A comprehensive risk assessment should include questions about current levels of risk as well as any historically presenting (in the past) risk for the YP in question.

Anna Dagnall is a specialist lecturer on CWP, EMHP, and HICBT programmes, an experienced clinical supervisor, and a CBT therapist. Anna highlights that risk is dynamic in nature, meaning that it can change, and emphasises the importance of exploring risk collaboratively and compassionately with YP. She says,

> Risk should always be considered in the context of the YP's life and the systems they have around them, such as family, school, or their community. Drawing on this can help manage any current or future risk, working with trusted adults who can support them outside of the CWP sessions.

Identifying protective factors, including positive relationships, helpful activities and interests, hopes for the future, and a desire for change, is a helpful place to start in developing a risk management plan. Even where there is an absence of any identified risk for a YP, having a risk management (or "staying safe") plan in place is good practice. This may be as straightforward as asking a YP what they would do, or who they would talk to, if things changed or they did feel at risk in any way. Best practice is to provide a written copy of such a plan to the YP or family, and it is imperative to always effectively document risk assessment and management in case notes.

Routine Outcome Measurement

To support information gathered in the assessment, you will make use of questionnaires called ROMs. These questionnaires generally produce a numeric (quantitative) score. This can then be interpreted, using predetermined cut-off scores or thresholds, to help understand how much of a problem a YP is experiencing.

For example, a YP's answers to the questions might give them a low score, under the cut-off point, indicating that it is unlikely they are having a significant difficulty or problem in that area (such as low mood, generalised anxiety, or panic). They may have a higher score in a different area, that is over the cut-off point, meaning that they possibly or probably (depending on how high the score is) have a clinically relevant difficulty in that area.

The questionnaires can be completed by children and YP, by their parents or carers, and, in some cases, by teachers also. There are different types of questionnaires available, with some aimed at different age ranges or with different purposes (such as finding out what the main problem is, finding out how they're feeling this week, or asking how the young person has found the session with a CWP). Lots of information about ROMs can be found on the Child Outcome Research Consortium website – www.corc.uk.net.

As a CWP, you will be trained to make use of a specific range of ROMs that are in line with your work and suitable for the population you are working with (i.e., children and YP). Collection of the data from these ROMs can be done at an individual level, to support the specific case, but can also be reviewed at a service level or a national level to get an overview of the effectiveness of the work being done and the impact on children, YP, and families.

When data is collected nationally, this is done via the NHS minimum data set (MDS). In the adult PP world, what CWPs would refer to as ROMs tend to be called MDS – this demonstrates how language can differ across the roles even where the practice is very similar.

Commonly used ROMs within assessment include the following:

- Revised Child Anxiety and Depression Scale (RCADS)
  This is a 47-item self-report questionnaire, used for ages 8–18 years. There is a YP version and a parent/carer version. Scoring is given under categories of separation anxiety disorder, social phobia, generalised anxiety disorder (GAD), panic disorder, obsessive compulsive disorder, and low mood (or major depressive disorder).

  You may also use RCADS subscales (i.e., a shorter version which just asks the questions relevant to one of the categories listed above) to carry on checking in on that single area across the course of an intervention.

  It is important to note that although the word disorder is included in the naming of these categories, this ROM is not diagnostic, meaning that a diagnosis cannot be made based upon it. CWPs are not trained to give YP a diagnosis.

- Strengths and Difficulties Questionnaire (SDQ)
  This is a 25-item emotional and behavioural screening questionnaire that can be self-completed by YP aged 11–17 years. There are also parent/carer and teacher versions that can be used for children aged between 2 and 17 years. The SDQ gives scoring under the five categories of emotional symptoms, conduct problems, hyperactivity/inattention, peer relationship problems, and prosocial behaviour.

When making use of ROMs, it is important to try and balance the different ways in which they can be useful. As explained above, they can be useful for you (the practitioner) in understanding the problem, as well as being useful for the service to understand the impact. They should also be used in a way that is helpful and meaningful to the YP or family being supported. The 'sweet spot' for ROM use is being able to capture all these elements, as shown in Figure 4.1.

Georgina Shires is a specialist lecturer on CWP, EMHP, Supervisor, and SWP programmes, an experienced clinical supervisor and CBT therapist, and passionate about the use of ROMs. She says "ROMs are integral in hearing the YP's voice. They can be used measure changes in symptoms, see improvement, and to facilitate conversations with YP and families in a meaningful way".

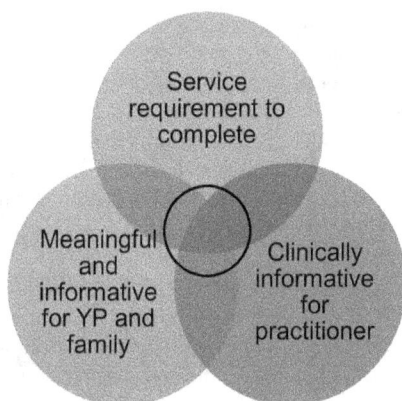

Figure 4.1 Meaningful Use of ROMs.

Shared Decision-Making

Once information about the presenting problem has been gathered in an assessment, and a thorough risk assessment has been conducted, the next step is for you to give information on what options for support are available. This then allows the YP, and their parent or carer if appropriate, to make choices about what type of support they would like, or even if they would like to carry on and access support at all.

There may be cases where sharing the details of what is happening for a YP, having someone (you, a lovely CWP, for example!) hear, validate, and make sense of their experience, and knowing that there is a reason their thoughts, feelings, and actions (behaviours) are linked together can be enough for some YP and families. They may choose not to continue and access any further support, and this is an ok outcome from the assessment as well.

However, in most cases, assessment will lead on to some kind of support being recommended and put in place for the YP. With LI CBT, and the brief nature of support, it is important that the YP is on board with the plan. If they are engaged in accessing support, they are more likely to complete between-session tasks (sometimes referred to as homework or home tasks), which will enhance what is completed within the CWP sessions.

It may sometimes be appropriate following an assessment for you to tell the YP and family that you will seek advice first and then get back to offer options for support. This then gives time for the case to be taken to clinical supervision and discussed. However, wherever possible, the YP and family should be given a clear understanding of when and how they will hear back from you (such as via phone call or via letter within a specific time period). This supports their involvement in decisions around what to do next.

Part of the process of shared decision-making is coming to a clear understanding of the problem together, as practitioner and YP or family. This is sometimes called formulation. As a PP, you might begin to formulate the problem yourself, discuss formulation in supervision, and then present your formulation (understanding of the problem) back to the YP or family to check they agree with it. The information you have gathered, problem analysis or RIA, and ROM scores will all be considered as part of this. Sometimes models, such as a 5 areas or thoughts-feelings-behaviour model, will be used to visually present information in a formulation.

Signposting

Signposting, which involves identifying and supporting YP and families to access services other than those of the CWP, can be a large part of the role. As a front-line practitioner with a focus on early intervention, you may often be the first mental health or PP that a family meets. This might mean a significant proportion of cases where the thoroughly conducted CWP assessment identifies that CWP support is not the evidence-based or recommended intervention. You will therefore, instead of working directly with the YP or family yourself, draw upon knowledge of local services and provision and help direct to the more appropriate type of support.

Signposting can be used in cases where LI PP support is not suitable, for example, if the presenting need is more severe, or the evidence base indicates that HI therapy or a different modality is required.

It may also be appropriate to signpost if a YP's difficulty is determined not to be a mental health problem and instead might be related to physical health, neurodivergence, or even a social context-based problem. Signposting in these cases may be to a primary care service, neurodevelopmental pathway or support, or a youth work or social care-based support.

Interventions

Core interventions offered by CWPs and EMHPs are the same, due to the evidence base, as well as overlapping core modules 1–3 on the respective curricula (with modules 4–6 being where the courses diverge to cover specialisms in community-based or education-based working). More details on modules can be found towards the end of this chapter and in Chapter 8 – Being a Trainee. However, due to the overlap, the intervention content across the two chapters in this book is remarkably similar.

There have been some case examples provided by CWPs and EMHPs to illustrate the overview of interventions. If you particularly benefit from the case examples to support your understanding, you may wish to read both chapters to capture as much of this content as possible.

General Principles of Working

There are some general principles or ways of working you will use, regardless of the specific intervention being offered. Some of these are as follows:

- Collaborative working – this is best described as 'doing with rather than doing to' and is the principle of working alongside the YP and giving them choice and control over the sessions where it is possible.
- Agenda setting – you will set an agenda, to-do list, or list of tasks, at the start of every session to guide what will be covered and ensure the YP knows what to expect. This agenda should be set in a collaborative way with the YP, allowing them to add items that they want to cover, and giving them some choice in order or timings of items where possible.
- Home tasks – CWP intervention work will be supported outside of the session by home tasks (sometimes called homework, but we know YPs don't always like this term!) These will help the YP practice new skills and start to make changes, often with

support from an identified adult (commonly a parent). Home tasks from the previous week will be reviewed at each session also, to see how the YP has gotten on.
- Goal-based working – making use of goals to aim towards with CWP sessions means that progress can be checked along the way, and there is a clear direction to the work completed.

Risk

Anna Dagnall (who we met earlier in this chapter) reminds us, "Risk trumps everything!". Risk should be reviewed at every session you offer, to check if anything has changed since the YP was last seen, and make sure that any risk management plan that has been developed is still suitable.

Anna tells us, "If something related to risk comes up during a treatment session, then the session content should be paused. You can come back to the intervention another time, but risk *must* be managed first".

Anna's advice is relevant whether risk is discovered by you asking about it, through general conversation, through the YP choosing to share, or any other means. This is part of the duty of care you hold as a PP.

Behavioural Activation

You will be trained to deliver BA as an intervention for low mood or depression. BA is an intervention that can be utilised within LI CBT, where it is considered a stand-alone treatment, and is also a component intervention of HICBT treatment. There is a substantial evidence base supporting the effectiveness of BA, with research with adults showing that the LI delivery of BA can be as effective as its use within a broader HICBT treatment.

BA as an intervention is based upon the behavioural theory of depression. This considers that where depression presents, whether a trigger for the onset of this can be identified or not, it is kept going (maintained) by reinforcement of the depressed behaviour (the things the person does now they are depressed, such as spending more time alone or avoiding friends) and a lack of, or reduction in, reinforcement for the non-depressed behaviour (what they person was doing before they became depressed, such as engaging in hobbies or activities, or seeing friends and socialising).

Box 4.2   BA case example

An example of a low mood case from practice has been provided by a CWP, who will remain unnamed to preserve the anonymity of the YP they supported. The case example below is fully anonymised and makes use of a pseudonym, Mia, which is not the YP's real name.

Mia, age 13 years, had spent some time in the hospital for a physical health condition, and because of this, she had missed quite a lot of school, seen her friends a lot less, and stopped some of the activities she had previously enjoyed. Although Mia's physical health had improved and she had been discharged from the hospital, this experience had understandably left her feeling frustrated, low in mood, and somewhat hopeless.

Mia spoke with a CWP and explained that she had thoughts such as "I'm never going to feel better again" and "I can't be bothered getting out of bed". She felt tired and fatigued, which made it harder to get back to doing the things she had done before. Mia also sometimes worried about her physical health deteriorating again and being in pain again, which also kept her from doing things.

As a result of how she felt, Mia was withdrawing further from her family and friends, spending more time alone in her bedroom, and leaving the house much less than she used to before she had been in the hospital.

BA as an intervention addresses low mood or depression by gradually increasing activity and opportunity for non-depressed behaviours to be re-established, so that reinforcement of these can be experienced. It is a behavioural intervention, making changes to what a person *does* in order to modify how they think and feel, rather than addressing the thinking first (as in a cognitive intervention). This makes it appropriate for a LI PP to effectively deliver, with evidence and research backing this up.

Early stages of this intervention will involve collecting information about what a YP is doing currently and what their days look like, whilst they are feeling low in mood. An activity diary, or activity log, is a method of recording what they are doing, even if this is what they might describe as doing 'nothing', such as lying in bed, scrolling their phone, or sleeping. Activity monitoring in this way is often used for this intervention as a between-session home task. Reviewing the information brought back by YP will then allow for curious conversations and the beginning of a plan to introduce new activity.

When planning a new activity, it can be beneficial to pick things that match a YP's values, the things that matter to them. Susan Moore, a qualified CWP, explains that this is one of the elements of the intervention she particularly likes because it introduces the YPs back to themselves. This intervention allows you and YP to start from scratch or 'hit the refresh button', identifying the YP's values together, and the 'key ingredients' that allow them to thrive.

Once new activities are introduced, you will support the YP to reflect on how this impacts their mood, consider building on the activities, and plan for increasing activity further going forward in a balanced way. You can act as a supportive, 'coaching', and motivating person to the YP at this stage, reinforcing any changes made through praise and encouragement.

Box 4.3   BA case example continued

The case example of Mia is continued below, again fully anonymised and making use of a pseudonym.

After exploring the problem with Mia, her CWP was able to support her to work through a BA intervention. Mia was able to add in some, initially small, activities that she had previously enjoyed, and in time noticed that this was helping her to feel better. She was able to socialise with her friends more and spend more time with her family, instead of on her own in her bedroom.

Mia's CWP helped her to consider her physical health needs alongside this increased activity, so that it felt manageable for her. Mia said that she felt 'heard and understood' by the CWP and that the support given had been really helpful for her.

Many CWP courses around the country utilise a specific manualised approach to BA, known as Brief Behavioural Activation (Brief BA) (Pass & Reynolds, 2021). This manualised approach has been clinically trialled, giving it a robust evidence base. It has been developed to include handouts for YP and parents to support each session, which are all available within a book that acts as a practitioner manual and guide. These resources make it popular with trainees and qualified CWPs alike.

Worry Management

Where problematic worry (sometimes referred to as generalised anxiety, or GAD if diagnostic criteria are met) is the identified presenting problem for a YP, you can offer WM. This intervention is behavioural in nature and can be useful for helping YP where the *act* (or behaviour) of worrying is the main thing getting in the way of day-to-day life and things they would rather be doing.

Charlotte Temple, a specialist lecturer on CWP, EMHP, Supervisor, SWP, and HICBT programmes, a clinical supervisor, and an experienced CBT therapist, has a keen interest in WM for LI practitioners (CWPs and EMHPs). Charlotte says

In practice WM will often be one of the most frequent interventions used by CWPs and EMHPs. The key point of the intervention is around helping YP manage the process of worrying itself, moving away from the content of worry thoughts.

This approach, managing worry as a behaviour, fits with the behavioural approach offered by CWPs, whilst supporting YP in managing their worries in a different way. YP who are 'worriers' (and this is often the way YP who experience problematic worry have been described) are often used to trying to address each individual worry as it comes along. They may do this in a variety of ways, common methods including seeking reassurance from others, preparing for things an excessive amount, making lots of very detailed plans, or simply spending a lot of time worrying about it. There is often a belief that worrying is helpful and will prevent the worst from happening.

This intervention will spend very little time on exploring the content of individual worries. It can be useful to know a little bit

about what types of worries YP have, as this supports implementing some of the new WM techniques, but the individual
worries won't be addressed. This can be a surprise to some YP.
Instead, the intervention addresses the behaviour or process of
worry and supports YP to change what they do about their
worries.

Box 4.4 WM case example

*An example of a WM case from practice has been provided
by a CWP, who will remain unnamed to preserve the anonymity of the YP they supported. The case example below
is fully anonymised and makes use of a pseudonym, Joel,
which is not the YP's real name.*

Joel, age 17 years, was experiencing 'constant worry'
about 'everything' in his life, with his upcoming exams and
the future as particular themes. He would have thoughts like
"What if I don't get the grades I need", despite doing well at
school, and "What if my parents are upset or disappointed",
despite their regular reassurance that they just wanted him
to 'be happy'. Joel explained to his CWP that he sometimes
even worried "about not worrying enough!" Joel felt regularly stressed, 'awful', and upset, and when particularly
worried described feeling like he would be sick, his heart
would beat fast, and his hands would get sweaty.

Joel would spend a lot of time revising but said he
didn't feel like he was getting anything done. Sometimes,
he would sit at his desk 'just worrying' instead. Joel sometimes avoided his friends because of how he felt, not
responding to their messages. However, he felt that this
would make him worry more about if his friends would
stop liking him.

Supporting YP to identify the type of worry they are experiencing is one of the first steps in WM. The types of worry are generally categorised as 'real' or 'hypothetical'; however, many CWPs
choose to adjust the language here to be more child-friendly.

Amelia Bellmon is an associate lecturer on CWP and EMHP programmes, qualified as a CWP and HICBT therapist, and an experienced LI clinical supervisor. Amelia says,

> Using the world real to describe one type of worry could potentially lead a YP to think we're saying that the other type of worry, hypothetical worries, aren't real, and this could feel quite invalidating. I prefer to use the term 'problem solvable worries' instead of 'real'. I also find the word hypothetical isn't very child friendly, so I call those worries 'what if worries'. If a YP has a different way of describing them, then I'd use their own language too.

Once the YP understands the two different types of worry, they can practice sorting their worries. There are then different ways of dealing with each type of worry. If the worry is 'real' (or 'problem solvable'), then a problem-solving technique can be taught and utilised. This involves helping the YP list all the possible things that could be done in response to the problem, identify what is good and bad about each option, and then choose the best option to try out, scheduling in a time to do this and who might be needed to help them with it.

If the worry is 'hypothetical' (or a 'what if worry'), then the YP is supported to recognise this and understand that there isn't anything they can do to change whether the worry will happen or not. They can then make use of 'let it go' techniques to take their mind off the worry. You may spend time helping the YP develop their own range of 'let it go' techniques, finding out what is most helpful for them.

One final element of WM is working on tolerance of uncertainty. YPs who worry tend to dislike uncertainty, in part because uncertainty can give lots of space for hypothetical or 'what if' worries to take over. Situations that are uncertain are often managed by trying to create more certainty, through preparing, asking lots of questions, or only doing certain things (avoiding those things that are very uncertain). However, the problem with this is that life is often uncertain, and absolute certainty is hard to achieve, particularly if you want to go about your life and enjoy it.

Tolerating uncertainty work involves supporting YP to change their behaviour around uncertainty (again, sticking with a behavioural approach that fits with the CWP role), so that, instead of creating more certainty, they can get used to being ok with some uncertainty. This is done in a similar way to a graded exposure intervention (read on in this chapter for more details on this intervention). This involves trying out easier steps towards uncertainty first and gradually getting more used to it and how it feels. Charlotte Temple (who we met earlier in the chapter) highlighted to us the effectiveness of this element and how well it can fit with an LI behaviour-based approach to WM.

Graded Exposure

Graded exposure can be offered for anxiety presentations where avoidance is a key factor in keeping the problem going (maintenance). Presentations appropriate for this intervention might include specific phobia, separation anxiety, symptoms of panic (subthreshold for panic disorder) or anxiety with a social element, and related avoidance behaviours (not meeting diagnostic criteria for social phobia).

Box 4.5   Graded exposure case example

An example of an exposure case from practice has been provided by a CWP, who will remain unnamed to preserve the anonymity of the YP they supported. The case example below is fully anonymised and makes use of a pseudonym, Imani, which is not the YP's real name.

Imani, age 11 years, was experiencing lots of worry and anxiety in relation to situations where she may have to do something, or speak to someone, alone. Examples of these situations included going to get something in the shop for their Mum or ordering food when eating out.

Imani told her CWP that thoughts such as "What if someone talks to me?" or "What if I can't find it (the item for Mum) and have to ask for help?" will go through their mind. She will feel stressed and scared, and notices that her stomach 'drops', she feels sick, a bit sweaty, and her heart pounds. Imani will usually ask Mum if she really must do it (whatever the task is) by herself and will try to refuse and avoid it if she can. If Mum insists, then Imani will take her sister with her as support.

Graded exposure is based on supporting the YP to have gradually increasing amounts of contact with the object or situation causing anxiety. Rebecca Sommerville-Clegg, a qualified CWP, tells us she likes this intervention because "It provides a safe space for young people to address and work on their fears when they are ready to do so".

Having identified the YP's anxiety-inducing object (e.g., dog) or situation (e.g., speaking to someone they don't know), you will support a YP to build a list of examples of related things that would make them feel anxious. These can then be rated and ordered, so that the result is a list from the least anxiety-provoking example to the most anxiety-provoking example. Rating can be done using a number, from 0 to 10, or a percentage, from 0 to 100%.

Where possible, there should be enough things on the list to gradually work up, without too big a jump in the level of anxiety. For example, if a YP has a dog phobia, watching a video of a dog jumping and barking might create anxiety that YP rates as three out of ten. However, walking across a field where dogs are running around off the lead might create anxiety rated as ten out of ten. This is obviously a large jump, so it would be helpful for you to support YP to fill in the gaps. Finding other examples of things that give some anxiety, at ratings in between three and ten, helps ensure that the exposure is graded and more likely to be successful.

The content of the exposure sessions would include supporting the YP to have contact with things from their list. Lists are sometimes drawn out as steps or ladders, with the term for this being a hierarchy. Rebecca Sommerville-Clegg (who we met earlier) says, "The ladder enables CWPs and YP to work together, taking the steps needed for that YP to overcome anxiety".

To get the best outcome from exposure, you support YP to really focus on the task, without using distractions or avoidance techniques (such as thinking of something else or not looking directly at the object). Across sessions, you will help the YP work their way up the ladder, gradually getting used to contact with the object or situation causing them anxiety and developing new learning that they can manage it and will be ok.

Box 4.6   Graded exposure case example continued

The case example of Imani is continued below, again fully anonymised and making use of a pseudonym.

After getting a clear understanding of what situations caused anxiety for Imani, and being clear that the avoidance of social interactions didn't meet the criteria for social anxiety disorder (which would have meant needing to refer Imani on for more HI support, in line with recommendations and the evidence base), exposure work was able to begin.

Imani worked with her CWP to build a ladder of situations she would currently avoid, from the 'least scary' at the bottom up to the 'scariest' at the top. Working their way up the steps on the ladder helped Imani to learn that she could do things, even if they initially felt hard and brought on some anxiety, and the worst fears she thought of generally didn't happen.

Imani was able to reach a point in the exposure work where she could try things out with less planning (e.g., if a situation naturally arose where she might have to speak to someone, she would have a go instead of avoiding it), which she was pleased to tell her CWP about.

By the end of the intervention, Imani's anxiety levels had significantly decreased in all areas of her life, and she was discharged from the service feeling more positive overall.

Within this intervention, it is fully acknowledged that doing exposure steps and encountering something that makes you anxious isn't always easy – we wanted to be clear that we recognise this! Therefore, it is even more important to make the steps manageable and start with things that are low level, to support YP to experience success early on and be able to build on this as steps become trickier. Having an end goal in sight and ensuring that the YP is on board with wanting things to be different also helps.

Parent-Led Anxiety

You will be trained not only to work with children and YP directly but also to offer support via parents or carers. For clarity of writing purposes, we will continue this section using the term 'parent'; however, we would like to make clear that any adult who has regular and primary care responsibility for a child can be appropriate for this support. This might include, but is not limited to, birth, step, or adoptive parents, grandparents, or other adult family members with a direct care responsibility for the child, foster carers, kinship carers, and more.

This type of support is sometimes referred to as 'parenting work', or parent-led CBT. There is strong evidence to demonstrate that working via parents is effective, particularly with children of primary school age.

This work to support parents is obviously a distinct difference from the PWP or MHWP role. EMHPs and CWPs will often spend considerable time interacting with parents, carers, and other adults in the systems supporting children and YP.

Lisa Buffel, a qualified CWP, backs the benefits of parent work from her own experience delivering this intervention. She says,

> Having parents directly involved in support has been proven, both by the evidence base and by experience in delivering the intervention, to significantly improve outcomes, as well as strengthening the parent-child relationship. I enjoy the opportunity to work with parents. It's great to see their knowledge around anxiety, as well as their confidence, grow.

For children of primary age presenting with anxiety difficulties, including generalised anxiety, separation anxiety, or phobias, you are taught to deliver a parent-led CBT-informed approach supported by a book, *Helping Your Child with Fears and Worries* (Creswell & Willetts, 2019), which parents work through alongside support.

The approach, which has been clinically trialled for effectiveness, is designed as a combination of face-to-face and telephone-based support. This can improve access for parents who may have other responsibilities and competing demands on their time. Support is delivered directly to the parent, or parents, with the child generally not attending the sessions. The only exception to this is the assessment session, where it can be beneficial to meet the child and ensure that their voice is included in gathering of information on the problem.

The intervention itself is based around taking a stepped, or graded, method to challenging fear and worry and supporting parents to develop a 'have a go' approach alongside their child. The underpinning theory is called exposure and inhibitory learning, which means supporting the child or young person to 'have a go' and encounter the thing that they would usually avoid due to anxiety, so that they can learn that the outcome they are afraid of doesn't usually happen, or if it does – they can cope with it!

Parent-Led Behaviour

A second intervention delivered directly to a parent or carer is the parent-led intervention for low-level problems with behaviour. This intervention is designed to support parents and carers of children aged 10 years and under and, as with the previously described parent-led intervention, has strong evidence for its effectiveness.

Gareth Edwards is a specialist lecturer on CWP and EMHP programmes, a CBT therapist, and experienced in supporting parents and families. Gareth acknowledges that talking about parenting can be emotive and tells us, "It is not uncommon for practitioners to feel that they are insensitively or clumsily prying when completing an assessment and gathering information about the problem". He shares that holding onto the core competencies of practice, such as curiosity and collaboration, while consistently giving clarity on the practitioner's role and remit, and why you are asking the questions you are, can help manage this.

The intervention is designed to support parents of children, between 2 and 9 years old, presenting with mild problems with their behaviour. These problems should not meet clinical thresholds or criteria for diagnosable disorders, such as Conduct Disorder, defined within the Diagnostic and Statistical Manual of Mental Disorders, Fifth Edition (APA, 2013).

The intervention emphasises broad principles of parenting and enhances parenting strategies, rather than prescribing specific techniques. It aims to prevent escalation of problem behaviours, meaning that it is a preventative intervention in fitting with the remit of CWPs. Gathering information on specific problem behaviours at the assessment stage is important and can be effectively done by the use of curious questioning and exploring a recent incident (via RIA). As with all PP work, parents are supported to set goals to work towards, identifying what they would like to be different and what they would hope to achieve via support.

The intervention is split into two broad sections, with the first focusing on promoting and enhancing the parent–child relationship and the second including routines, boundaries, and limit setting. Across the early sessions, you will support the parent to understand their child's current behaviour and what might impact on this, in fitting with CBT-informed approaches and psychoeducation.

You will then support the parent to introduce time for focused play with their child, sometimes referred to as 'special time', with emphasis on this being child-led. A nice metaphor that can be used to explain the rationale for this can be that of putting money into a piggy bank to invest. In a similar way, spending positive time together is explained as investing in the relationship and their child.

Following this, you will work with the parent on making use of more regular and specific praise with their child. Research shows that where children are praised in a way that is specific, such as "you've really taken your time with that picture, well done", as opposed to more generic or outcome-focused, such as "you're excellent at drawing", it can increase motivation and positively influence self-esteem and self-evaluation.

The later sessions include supporting the parent to manage unwanted behaviours through strategies such as improving boundaries and expectations, giving effective commands, withdrawing attention (i.e., not responding) when unwanted behaviours are displayed, using calm time, and enforcing consequences when boundaries are crossed.

It is important to clarify that, within strategies for enforcing consequences, there is strong emphasis on promoting non-violent and non-punitive discipline approaches. It is also important to be clear that withdrawing attention may not be possible if a child is behaving in a way that is dangerous or destructive. In these instances, the use of calm time and/or consequences may be unavoidable, so this is discussed with parents and planned for.

One of the key methods utilised in parent-led interventions, with strong evidence for its effectiveness, is brought in here. Modelling and rehearsal are experiential learning methods that support parents to 'have a go' and practice skills and strategies before going home to try them with their child. This means, in a general sense, that you and the parent practice (sometimes called 'role play', but we acknowledge this word can put people off) within the session, one person 'being' the child and one 'being' the parent.

At some points, the parent might be best placed to be the child, so they can give examples of what their child might say, and you will 'be' the parent, so you can demonstrate (model) new strategies and ways of responding. At other points, you might take on the role of the child, so that the parent can 'be' themself and practice different strategies and responses.

Gareth Edwards (who we met earlier) highlights the benefits of collaboration and teamwork in parent interventions. He acknowledges,

> Many parents may begin the process somewhat pessimistically, due to their view of what the problem is and/or previous experiences of working with services. However, parents' knowledge, experience, and insight, coupled with the practitioner's approaches, and supported by an effective therapeutic relationship, can produce a really successful intervention and outcome.

Qualification and Changes

At the launch of the CWP role in 2017, the awarded qualification was a postgraduate certificate (PGCert) or graduate certificate, with 60 credits to be completed, generally split across three modules.

Modules were defined in the curriculum as follows:

Module 1: Children and YP's mental health settings: context and values

Module 2: Assessment and engagement

Module 3: Evidence-based interventions for common mental health problems with children and YP (theory and skills)

In 2023, changes were introduced, with developments made to the curriculum, and the awarded qualification became a post-graduate diploma or graduate diploma, with 120 credits to be completed. The curriculum adjustments added a further three modules to provide the additional 60 credits. The focus of these additional modules was on the elements of community working that would distinguish the CWP role from the EMHP role.

Additional modules as defined in the curriculum are as follows:

Module 4: Working, assessing, and engaging in community-based and primary care mental health service settings

Module 5: Mental health prevention in community and primary care settings

Module 6: Interventions for emerging mental health difficulties in community and primary health care settings

Ellie McKelvey is a current CWP trainee and told us, "I appreciate the move to the diploma as I feel we are getting a more rounded offer".

It should be noted that these are the modules as defined by the national curriculum, but there may be differences in naming and module breakdown across different higher education institutes or training providers. More detailed discussion of the qualifications can be found in Chapter 8 – Being a Trainee.

Community Specialist Role

With the changes made to the curriculum in 2023, the community working element of the CWP role was further embedded into training courses. There was always an intention for CWPs to work outside of traditional clinical settings and be based in community venues, from the very first year of the course. The original curriculum, for the PGCert included details such as "the primary objective is to facilitate access to support from community services, reduce waiting lists to wider CYPMH services, offer evidence-based help to children and YP with mild to moderate difficulties" and "the CWP role will deliver significant elements of their contribution in the context of other community agencies or 'platforms'".

The CWP curriculum identifies that you should work within community and primary care settings and goes on to further describe this as including voluntary community services, charities, primary health care providers, religious and social groups, and civic institutions that communities use. Pretty much anywhere that YP spend time when not at home or in school, or indeed when they are not accessing school. In practice, this may mean that you are working via settings such as GP surgeries, health centres, child and family centres, youth clubs, faith settings, and so on.

As well as aims for you to offer core assessments and interventions within these settings, there are also new elements of working established for CWPs in community settings. These elements include engagement activities with community organisations, delivery of training to staff in community settings, delivery of psychoeducation to children, YP, parents, carers, and staff, and groupwork delivery to YP or parents in community settings.

Rebecca Sommerville-Clegg, a qualified CWP we met earlier in this chapter, tells us about her community-based work.

> I attend community events for services and charities in the area my team is based. This allows me to meet with other professionals and families to promote the benefits of looking after ourselves and our mental health and introduce my team and service. I can offer support for children, YP, and families in a way that is outside of education or a clinic setting.

Rebecca also notes the benefits for her own practice, saying, "By engaging in the local community I also learn more about the services in my area, that I can then refer families to for support if they need something other than I can offer".

Conclusion

We hope that this chapter has given you a good insight into the CWP role and what this can look like in practice. Is this the PP role for you? If not, please read on to Chapter 5 for an overview of the EMHP role, or revisit Chapter 2 or 3 to learn about the adult roles of PWP and MHWP.

If the CWP role does sound like a good fit, then that's wonderful and welcome to the team – you may want to move on to Chapter 6 and beyond to continue exploring your career options.

Box 4.7   References and wider reading

American Psychiatric Association. (2013). *The diagnostic and statistical manual of mental disorders. 5th Edition*. American Psychiatric Association.

Creswell, C., & Willetts, L. (2019). *Helping your child with fears and worries. 2nd Edition*. Robinson.

Department of Health & NHS England. (2015). *Future in mind: Promoting, protecting, and improving our children and young people's mental health and wellbeing*. NHS England.

HM Government. (2011). *No health without mental health: A cross-government mental health outcomes strategy for people of all ages*.

Mental Health Taskforce. (2014). *Five year forward view*. NHS England.

Pass, L., & Reynolds, S. (2021). *Brief behavioural activation for adolescent depression: A clinician's manual and session-by-session guide*. Jessica Kingsley Publishers.

Wolpert, M., Harris, R., Hodges, S., Fuggle, P., James, R., & Wiener, A. (2019). *THRIVE framework for system change*. CAMHS Press.

Chapter 5

Being an Education Mental Health Practitioner

Introduction and Background

With the publication, in 2017, of *Transforming Children and Young People's Mental Health Provision: A Green Paper* (Department for Health & Department for Education), a new low-intensity psychological practitioner (PP) role was also introduced, the education mental health practitioner (EMHP). The aim of this role was to train practitioners who could work in newly developed Mental Health Support Teams (MHSTs). These MHSTs would be linked to groups of primary schools, secondary schools, and colleges in the locality area, providing interventions to children and young people (YP) who were experiencing mild to moderate common mental health (MH) difficulties.

As with the children's wellbeing practitioner (CWP) role, the EMHP role drew upon the experiences and success of the psychological wellbeing practitioner (PWP) role and the adult Improving Access to Psychological Therapies (IAPT) programme. In some ways, the EMHP shares more similarities with the PWP role than the CWP role does, in that both PWPs and EMHPs are designed to sit within purpose-designed services – National Health Service (NHS) Talking Therapies for Anxiety and Depression Step 2 services for the PWP and MHSTs for the EMHP. The structure provided by these services can support the effectiveness of the role, ensuring that early-intervention, preventative services are giving access to those who are recently presenting with difficulties or have not accessed MH support before.

The development of the EMHP role continued to expand the Children and Young People's IAPT programme, which had been

DOI: 10.4324/9781003542049-5

established in 2011. CYP IAPT was initially rolled out into existing Child and Adolescent Mental Health Services (CAMHS) teams as a service transformation programme. This meant that staff were being trained from within existing staff teams, developing their skills and competencies (be that in a high-intensity psychological therapy, supervision, or leadership), and enhancing the evidence-based offer from the service. This was different to the adult IAPT programme, where new services were developed at Step 2 to 'house' the newly trained staff and develop a new and distinct offer.

As already mentioned, the EMHP role and its structure of sitting within a purpose-developed MHST is a slight shift away from direct service transformation and moves closer to the design around the PWP role. MHSTs are in many cases housed under NHS Trusts and will link closely with CAMHS teams; however, they have a clear and distinct referral pathway.

The development of the CYP IAPT programme, which, in more recent years, has changed title to Children and Young People's Psychological Training (CYP PT), has included training in a range of therapies and therapeutic modalities over the years, including cognitive behavioural therapy (CBT), parent training, systemic family practice, and interpersonal therapy for adolescents, as well as the low-intensity PP roles.

This has all been underpinned by guidance and government publications such as *No Health without Mental Health: A Cross-Government Strategy* (2011), *The Five Year Forward View* (2014), *Future in Mind* (2015), the *Mental Health Taskforce Report* (2016), and the *Green Paper* (2017) mentioned at the beginning of this chapter.

These publications outlined, amongst other things, the need for a significant expansion of the workforce in the Children and Young People's Mental Health Service (CYPMHS), to close the gap between what was needed (the demand) and what evidence-based support was available (the provision). They also gave recommendations on what needed to be done to improve the ways in which children's MH and wellbeing could be supported, highlighting that, when ill, children and Y should receive good quality and timely care. The *Green Paper*, in particular, made links between this need for increased early MH support and preventative work and the role of the education sector.

Box 5.1 Quote from the *Green Paper*

"This green paper builds on Future in Mind and the ongoing expansion of NHS-funded provision, and sets out our ambition to go further to ensure that children and YP showing early signs of distress are always able to access the right help, in the right setting, when they need it.

We know that half of all mental health conditions are established before the age of fourteen, and we know that early intervention can prevent problems escalating and have major societal benefits. Informed by widespread existing practice in the education sector and by a systematic review of existing evidence on the best ways to promote positive mental health for children and YP, we want to put schools and colleges at the heart of our efforts to intervene early and prevent problems escalating".

Transforming Children and Young People's Mental Health Provision: A Green Paper (2017)

The trailblazer (pilot) cohorts of EMHPs began training in 2018. The training places are often recruited to train positions, meaning that new staff are brought into the workforce for the purpose of training.

The CYP PT programme is underpinned by a set of principles for working. These were initially referred to as the CYP IAPT Principles, but, more recently, have become the CYP Psychological Training Principles, with the move away from the term IAPT. The five principles are as follows:

- **Accessibility**
  This involves increasing the amount of access for CYP and families to MH and wellbeing support.
- **Accountability**
  This encourages the use of outcome measurement (via routine outcome measures or ROMs) to hold services accountable for their work.
- **Awareness**
  This emphasises the need to increase awareness of MH issues and tackle stigma around mental ill-health in children and YP.

- **Evidence-Based Practice**
  This is a commitment to providing support and interventions that have a strong evidence base and keeping up to date with developments and changes in evidence.
- **Participation**
  This supports valuing and facilitating the active involvement of children, YP, parents, carers, and communities, at both an individual and a service level.

These principles are designed to work together, rather than independently, to ensure that they support and enhance the overall culture of CYPMH services.

An additional crucial aspect of the role of EMHP (and indeed all PP roles) is to ensure that all YP, parents, carers, and families are treated with respect and dignity, irrespective of any actual or perceived difference in characteristic, status, or element of their identity. This is often captured within terms such as cultural competency, cultural responsiveness, or equality, diversity, and inclusion. It is also incorporated into the codes of conduct and ethical practice for both registering bodies for PPs (the British Psychological Society and the British Association of Behavioural and Cognitive Psychotherapies).

There are a variety of ways that this can be put into practice by PPs, but, broadly, it means ensuring that the whole individual is seen within any assessment or intervention offered.

Grace Wiles and Jasmine Pugh are trainee EMHPs, working in the same MHST. They spoke to us about being aware of some communities in the area they work that tend not to access their service. They both felt that building awareness of the needs of this community and understanding the barriers' currently limiting access is an important part of culturally responsive working and an important part of their role.

Scope and Remit

The remit of an EMHP is to work with children and YP who are experiencing mild to moderate common MH difficulties, including anxiety, low mood, and behavioural difficulties. EMHPs can work directly with YP (where this is appropriately supported by the evidence base) or offer work with the parent or carer.

Work will be completed and referrals received via an education setting.

EMHPs are trained to comprehensively assess risk in all cases at the first point of contact and to check in on risk at each subsequent contact. However, it should be emphasised that the role is neither appropriate nor designed for the ongoing support of YP presenting with current risk to themselves or others, or significant levels of historic risk. The role is also not appropriate to support YP with serious or enduring MH problems or those requiring a more specialist level of care. EMHPs can offer early intervention for those with first incidence or recently presenting mild to moderate common MH difficulties, where a brief intervention is likely to make a difference.

Brief intervention generally means somewhere in the region of six to eight sessions of support, including an assessment within this. It may be that there are cases where fewer sessions are sufficient to achieve the identified goals for a YP, or where slightly more sessions are appropriate to offer (in a planned way).

As mentioned previously, and as clearly identified by the role title itself, the EMHP role is designed to work in education settings, which may include primary schools, secondary schools, colleges, and alternative education provision. As well as being identified in the *Green Paper*, this also ties in with the CYP PT principles of improving accessibility to evidence-based psychological treatment. EMHPs are also trained to offer support via remote methods, including telephone or online platforms such as MS Teams, Zoom, or service-specific secure platforms (not an exhaustive list).

EMHPs are trained to offer individual support, working one to one with YP or parents and carers. The key EMHP interventions of behavioural activation (BA), worry management (WM), and exposure (more details on these further on in this chapter) are all suitable for one-to-one support. However, it is crucial to note here that even where intervention is primarily offered one to one directly with a YP, we know that YPs have parents, carers, teachers, school pastoral staff, and wider support systems around them that must also be considered. This means that EMHPs, even when offering an individual intervention, will often include parents, carers, school staff, or other appropriate adults, in their sessions, or link these key adults in with the sessions via additional face-to-face contact or phone calls. The placement of EMHPs in education settings gives them improved access to these education staff to link them with interventions and support plans.

EMHPs can also offer group-based support, including delivery directly to YP or delivery to groups of parents and carers. Groups delivered by EMHPs will, in most cases, take place within the school setting, again increasing access to this type of support for those in the school community.

As well as offering these different types of direct intervention, the remit of an EMHP includes a significant element of assessment, followed up by signposting to other types of support. This will be discussed in more detail further in this chapter.

An element of support that is specific to the EMHP role is the delivery of Whole-School Approach (WSA) work. This work involves EMHPs working closely with allocated schools or colleges to prioritise and support the MH and wellbeing of the whole school or college community, with a set of eight core principles to guide. More details are given on WSA work further on in this chapter.

Population Served

EMHPs are trained to work with YP up to the age of 18 years, as well as with parents or carers directly. Referrals to EMHPs are made via the education settings to which they are linked, such as primary or secondary schools, colleges, or alternative education provision, and support will, in most cases, be offered within the education setting also.

Individual interventions may target specific age ranges in line with the supporting evidence base. For example, the Brief Behavioural Activation (Brief BA) manualised intervention (Pass & Reynolds, 2021) that is taught on many EMHP programmes is targeted specifically at adolescents. There are also specific age ranges identified for the taught parent-led interventions, where the evidence base supports working with parents instead of the child, generally up to 10 or 12 years.

Settings/Specified Systems of Care

The EMHP role is very specifically designed to work within an MHST. These teams can be set up and operated by NHS Trusts or via CYPMHS partnership organisations, such as charity providers of MH support.

In relation to the THRIVE Framework, a model for CYPMHS that has been rolled out across the past decade alongside wider CYP IAPT/CYP PT service transformation work, the EMHP role aligns most clearly to the 'Getting Advice' and 'Getting Help' quadrants. However, the role also supports the remaining areas of the model, 'Thriving', 'Getting More Help', and 'Getting Risk Support'. Further sources for reading on the Thrive model are included at the end of this chapter.

Where EMHPs are employed by NHS Trusts, they are paid at NHS Agenda for Change pay band 4 during their training year, rising to pay band 5 once qualified. Salaries in non-NHS organisations are generally broadly aligned to these rates of pay but may vary slightly.

It is important to note that a requirement of the EMHP role is that practitioners work within systems of care that provide appropriate pathways to further care where needed. This is often referred to as stepped care and ensures that EMHPs are not left holding cases that are outside the remit of their role, such as those with more severe MH difficulties needing more intensive psychological therapy or a wider package of care. This model of stepped care is in fitting with the design of the other PP roles (see Chapters 2–4 for further details).

A further specification of the systems in which EMHPs work is that there is appropriate clinical governance (which broadly means ways of checking practice and ensuring best outcomes for YP and families) and that accountability for professional practice is held by a senior member of staff. Within the MHSTs, these senior members of staff may be high-intensity cognitive behaviour therapists (HI CBT), clinical psychologists with CBT experience, or practitioners with other backgrounds who have experience and knowledge of CBT-informed practice and low-intensity CBT approaches.

We have also reached the stage in the lifespan of the EMHP role to allow qualified and experienced practitioners to complete further training as supervisors or senior wellbeing practitioners (SWPs – see Chapter 12 – Making the Most of Your Career for further details). This would then allow them to take on the senior role within the MHST and supervise the work of trainee or qualified EMHPs.

Clinical supervision is offered frequently for EMHPs and is distinct from line management supervision (LMS). Where LMS can generally be provided by anyone in a management position, clinical supervision must be provided by an appropriately qualified, experienced practitioner who usually also has training in CBT or CBT-informed practice.

Clinical supervision takes two forms:

- Clinical Case Management Supervision
  This is focused on reviewing the caseload of the EMHP. For qualified EMHPs, this should be offered at a minimum of one hour per fortnight and should be delivered individually.
- Clinical Skills Supervision
  This is focused on developing the skills of the EMHP. It is generally provided in a group format, with no more than four EMHPs in the group and a minimum of 30 minutes per practitioner. It should be offered at a minimum of one hour per fortnight for the first six months post-qualification, and thereafter a minimum of one hour per month.

Another key specification is that referral pathways to EMHPs should be directly from schools to the MHST and entirely distinct from existing referral routes to specialist CAMHS services. This ensures that cases being picked up by EMHPs for assessment are most likely to be suitable to receive a brief, low-intensity CBT-informed intervention, in line with the evidence base. Referrals received by EMHPs should be presenting with a primary problem of anxiety or low mood, with a recent onset of the problem, and minimal to no risk present.

Pre-Intervention

Assessment

Assessments conducted by EMHPs are based upon a CBT model, which means that the focus is on the here and now of the presenting problem. One of the aims is to identify the factors that are keeping the problem going, often referred to as maintenance factors. It can be beneficial to develop an understanding of the longer-term background of the YP who is seeking help (sometimes call a developmental history); however, this is not the primary goal of an EMHP assessment.

The principle underpinning CBT is that the thoughts an individual has will impact on how they feel, emotionally and physically, and this will, in turn, impact upon the things that they do (their behaviours). It is therefore key to a CBT-informed assessment to try and identify the thoughts, feelings (emotions and physical feelings in the body), and behaviours that are occurring in relation to the problem at hand.

You may ask a YP, or their parent or carer, to think of the most recent time they have experienced their presenting problem as a method of gathering information about the thoughts, feelings, and behaviours (TFB). Using a specific example can help the YP to more clearly recall what thoughts and feelings they may have had, and what they did as a result. Keeping it recent also makes this easier to do.

There are other techniques you may use to gather information. One of these is funnelling of questions, where a broad open question is asked first and then you 'funnel' down to further detail by using more specific and closed questions. You might also use Socratic questioning methods, which is a technique used in CBT that helps to guide a YP or parent to make their own links and develop their own understanding of the problem. Questioning techniques such as the 'W questions' (what, where, when, with whom, etc.) or FIDO (asking about frequency, intensity, duration, and onset of the problem) can also be utilised in gathering information.

When going into an assessment with a YP or parent/carer, you should always include an overview of confidentiality and the ways in which information about the YP will be recorded and stored. The best practice is to check with YPs what, if any, understanding they have of the word 'confidentiality' first, before then clarifying what it means and when information may not be able to be kept confidential (often referred to as 'breaking confidentiality'). It is important to do this at the start of the appointment, so that YP or parent/carers are aware of what might happen before they begin to share things with you.

As well as gathering information on the presenting problem, an initial assessment is a good opportunity for you to start to engage with the YP and build rapport. Asking about hobbies and interests, friendships, experience of school, and extra-curricular activity can give insight into the YP's life. Understanding who the YP has around them, in their family, living at home, and as a system of support, can also be part of this. Information obtained from teachers or key staff in schools may also enhance understanding of the YP.

You can use an activity such as creating a genogram, or family tree, to capture this information. This may also be an appropriate time to understand any difficult relationships the YP might have in their life. If parents are present in an assessment, they may also be able to provide an understanding of any MH difficulties in the family. This can be helpful as we know from research that some presenting difficulties may be more likely to occur where there are similar difficulties in other members of the family, as well as some behavioural elements of problems being reinforced (kept going) by others, or potentially learned vicariously (which means from others).

Risk assessment is an important part of an EMHP initial assessment, ensuring that risk is appropriately assessed and managed the first time a practitioner has contact with a YP or family. A comprehensive risk assessment should include questions about current levels of risk as well as any historically presenting (in the past) risk for the YP in question.

Anna Dagnall is a specialist lecturer on CWP, EMHP, and HI CBT programmes, an experienced clinical supervisor, and a CBT therapist. Anna highlights that risk is dynamic in nature, meaning that it can change, and emphasises the importance of exploring risk collaboratively and compassionately with YP. She says,

> Risk should always be considered in the context of the YP's life and the systems they have around them, such as family, school, or their community. Drawing on this can help manage any current or future risk, working with trusted adults who can support them outside of the EMHP sessions.

Identifying protective factors, including positive relationships, helpful activities and interests, hopes for the future, and a desire for change, is a helpful place to start in developing a risk management plan. Even where there is an absence of identified risk for a YP, having a risk management (or "staying safe") plan in place is good practice. This may be as straightforward as asking a YP what they would do, or who they would talk to, if things changed or they did feel at risk in any way. Best practice is to provide a written copy of such a plan to the YP or family, and it is imperative to always effectively document risk assessment and management in case notes.

Routine Outcome Measurement

To support information gathered in the assessment, you will make use of questionnaires called ROMs. These questionnaires generally produce a numeric (quantitative) score. This can then be interpreted, using predetermined cut-off scores or thresholds, to help understand how much of a problem a YP is experiencing.

For example, a YP's answers to the questions might give them a low score, under the cut-off point, indicating that it is unlikely they are having a significant difficulty or problem in that area (such as low mood, generalised anxiety, or panic). They may have a higher score in a different area, that is over the cut-off point, meaning that they possibly or probably (depending on how high the score is) have a clinically relevant difficulty in that area.

You will be trained to make use of a specific range of ROMs that are in line with your work and suitable for the population you are working with (i.e., children and YP). Collection of the data from these ROMs can be done at an individual level, to support the specific case (as described above), but can also be reviewed at a service level or a national level to get an overview of the effectiveness of the work being done and the impact on children, YP, and families.

When data is collected nationally, this is done via the NHS minimum data set (MDS). In the adult PP world, what EMHPs would refer to as ROMs tend to be called MDS – this demonstrates how language can differ across the roles even where the practice is very similar.

Commonly used ROMs within assessment include the following:

- Revised Child Anxiety and Depression Scale (RCADS)
  This is a 47-item self-report questionnaire that can be used for ages 8–18 years. There is a YP version and a parent/carer version. Scoring is given under the categories of separation

anxiety disorder, social phobia, generalised anxiety disorder (GAD), panic disorder, obsessive compulsive disorder, and low mood (or major depressive disorder).

EMHPs may also use RCADS subscales (i.e., a shorter version which just asks the questions relevant to one of the categories listed above) to carry on checking in on that single area across the course of an intervention.

It is important to note that although the word disorder is included in the naming of these categories, this ROM is not diagnostic, meaning that a diagnosis cannot be made based upon it. EMHPs are not trained to give YP a diagnosis.

• Strengths and Difficulties Questionnaire (SDQ)
This is a 25-item emotional and behavioural screening questionnaire that can be self-completed by YP aged 11–17 years. There are also parent/carer and teacher versions that can be used for children aged between 2 and 17 years. The SDQ gives scoring under the five categories of emotional symptoms, conduct problems, hyperactivity/inattention, peer relationship problems, and prosocial behaviour.

When making use of ROMs, it is important to try and balance the different ways in which they can be useful. As explained above, they can be useful for you, the practitioner, in understanding the problem, as well as being useful for the service to understand the

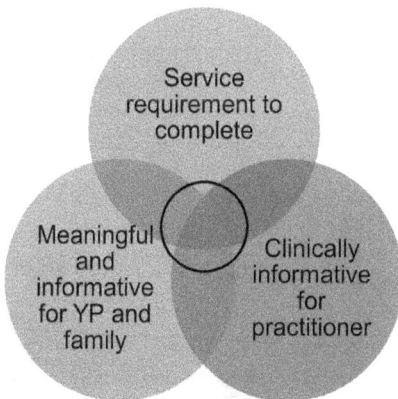

Figure 5.1 Meaningful Use of ROMs.

impact. They should also be used in a way that is helpful and meaningful to the YP or family being supported. The 'sweet spot' for ROM use is being able to capture all these elements, as shown in Figure 5.1.

Georgina Shires is a specialist lecturer on CWP, EMHP, Supervisor, and SWP programmes, an experienced clinical supervisor, and a CBT therapist, and is passionate about the use of ROMs. She says, "ROMs are integral in hearing the YP's voice. They can be used to measure changes in symptoms, see improvement, and to facilitate conversations with YP and families in a meaningful way".

Shared Decision-Making

Once information about the presenting problem has been gathered in an assessment, and a thorough risk assessment has been conducted, the next step is for you to give information on what options for support are available. This then allows the YP, and their parent or carer if appropriate, to make choices about what type of support they would like, or even if they would like to carry on and access support at all.

There may be cases where sharing the details of what is happening for a YP, having someone (you, a lovely EMHP, for example!) hear, validate, and make sense of their experience, and knowing that there is a reason their thoughts, feelings, and actions (behaviours) are linked together can be enough for some YP and families. They may choose not to continue and access any further support, and this is an ok outcome from an assessment.

However, in most cases, an assessment will lead on to some kind of support being recommended and put in place for the YP. With low-intensity CBT and the brief nature of support, it is important that the YP is on board with the plan. If they are engaged in accessing support, they are more likely to complete between-session tasks (sometimes referred to as homework or home tasks), which will enhance what is completed within the EMHP sessions.

It may sometimes be appropriate following assessment for you to tell the YP and family that they will seek advice first and then get back to offer options for support. This then gives time for the case to be taken to clinical supervision and discussed. However, wherever possible, the YP and family should be given a clear understanding of when and how they will hear back from you (such as in a follow-up appointment at school on a set date, via phone call, or via letter within a specific time period). This supports their involvement in decisions around what to do next.

Within an education setting, it may be appropriate for some feedback on the outcome of the assessment to be shared with the designated link person, who may be a member of staff in the pastoral team or a safeguarding lead. Where this is done, it is important to still maintain confidentiality for the YP and family, being sure that information shared is done so with appropriate consent.

Part of the process of shared decision-making is coming to a clear understanding of the problem together, as practitioner and YP or family. This is sometimes called formulation. As a PP, you might begin to formulate the problem yourself, discuss formulation in supervision, and then present your formulation (understanding of the problem) back to the YP or family to check they agree with it. The information you've gathered, problem analysis or RIA, and ROM scores will all be considered as part of this. Sometimes, models, such as a five areas or TFB model, will be used to visually present information in a formulation.

Signposting

Signposting, which involves identifying and supporting YP and families to access services other than those of the EMHP, can be a large part of the role. As a front-line practitioner with a focus on early intervention, you may often be the first MH or PP that a family meets. This might mean a significant proportion of cases where the thoroughly conducted EMHP assessment identifies that EMHP support is not the evidence-based or recommended intervention. You will therefore, instead of working directly with the YP or family themselves, liaise with the school link person and draw upon their knowledge of local services and provision to help direct the YP to a more appropriate type of support.

Signposting can be used in cases where low-intensity, PP support is not suitable, for example, if the presenting need is more severe, or the evidence base indicates that high-intensity therapy, or a different modality is required.

It may also be appropriate to signpost if a YP's difficulty is determined not to be an MH problem and, instead, might be related to physical health, neurodivergence, specific learning needs, or even a social context-based problem. Signposting in these cases may be to a primary care service, neurodevelopmental pathway or support, appropriate support within the school special educational needs and disabilities offer, or other support.

Interventions

Core interventions offered by CWPs and EMHPs are the same, due to the evidence base, as well as overlapping core modules 1–3 on the respective curricula (with modules 4–6 being where the courses diverge to cover specialisms in community-based or education-based working). More details on modules can be found towards the end of this chapter and in Chapter 8 – Being a Trainee. However, due to the overlap, the intervention content across the two chapters in this book is remarkably similar.

There have been some case examples provided by CWPs and EMHPs to illustrate the overview of interventions. If you particularly benefit from the case examples to support your understanding, you may wish to read both chapters to capture as much of this content as possible.

General Principles of Working

There are some general principles or ways of working used by EMHPs, regardless of the specific intervention being offered. Some of these are as follows:

- Collaborative working – this is best described as 'doing with rather than doing to' and is the principle of working alongside the YP and giving them choice and control over the sessions where it is possible.
- Agenda setting – you will set an agenda, to-do list, or list of tasks, at the start of every session to guide what will be covered and ensure the YP knows what to expect. This agenda should be set in a collaborative way with the YP, allowing them to add items that they want to cover, and giving them some choice in order or timings of items where possible.

- Home tasks – EMHP intervention work will be supported outside of the session by home tasks (sometimes called homework, but we know YP don't always like this term!) These will help the YP practice new skills and start to make changes, often with support from an identified adult (commonly a parent). Home tasks from the previous week will be reviewed at each session also, to see how the YP has gotten on.
- Goal-based working – making use of goals to aim towards with CWP sessions means that progress can be checked along the way, and there is a clear direction to the work completed.

Risk

Anna Dagnall (who we met earlier in this chapter) reminds us, "Risk trumps everything!". Risk should be reviewed at every session offered, to check if anything has changed since the YP was last seen and make sure that any risk management plan that has been developed is still suitable.

Anna tells us, "If something related to risk comes up during a treatment session, then the session content should be paused. You can come back to the intervention another time, but risk *must* be managed first".

Anna's advice is relevant whether risk is discovered by you asking about it, through general conversation, through the YP choosing to share, or any other means. This is part of the duty of care held by PPs.

Behavioural Activation

You will be trained to deliver BA as an intervention for low mood or depression. BA is an intervention that can be utilised within low-intensity CBT, where it is considered a stand-alone treatment, and is also a component intervention of HI CBT treatment. There is a substantial evidence base supporting the effectiveness of BA, with research with adults showing that the low-intensity delivery of BA can be as effective as its use within a broader HI CBT treatment.

BA as an intervention is based upon the behavioural theory of depression. This considers that where depression presents, whether a trigger for the onset of this can be identified or not, it is kept going (maintained) by reinforcement of the depressed behaviour (the things the person does now they are depressed, such as spending more time alone or avoiding friends) and a lack of, or reduction in, reinforcement for the non-depressed behaviour (what they person was doing before they became depressed, such as engaging in hobbies or activities, or seeing friends and socialising).

Box 5.2   BA case example from practice

An example of a low mood case from practice has been provided by an EMHP, who will remain unnamed to preserve the anonymity of the CYP they supported. The case example below is fully anonymised and makes use of a pseudonym, Sam, which is not the CYP's real name.

"Sam, age 15, had been feeling low in mood for several months, with no clear trigger to what had started this. Sam did not enjoy going to school anymore despite having a good circle of friends and would describe often coming home from school feeling tired and drained.

Sam explained to their EMHP that they would have thoughts like 'I don't have the energy to do anything as school is so tiring' and 'I'm letting everyone down', and this would cause them to worry that they would eventually lose their friends.

This led to Sam feeling low, helpless, frustrated, overwhelmed, and disconnected from those around them. Physically they were feeling fatigued, like their body was heavy and slowed down, they struggled to concentrate on lessons at school, and everything felt harder than usual.

As a result of how they were feeling, Sam was spending less time around their friends and opting out of any family activities. Their sleep pattern had changed, with them struggling to get to sleep at night and finding it hard to get up in the morning. Instead of engaging in activities and hobbies, they would spend hours on social media 'doom scrolling' or watching TV without really taking it in, as they didn't 'have the energy' for anything else. They explained that they were eating more junk food which made them feel worse too.

Overall, Sam was able to tell their EMHP that they didn't feel very hopeful about things improving".

BA as an intervention addresses low mood or depression by gradually increasing activity and opportunity for non-depressed behaviours to be re-established, so that reinforcement of these can be experienced. It is a behavioural intervention, making changes to what a person *does* in order to modify how they think and feel, rather than addressing the thinking first (as in a cognitive intervention). This makes it appropriate for a low-intensity PP to effectively deliver, with evidence and research backing this up.

Early stages of this intervention will generally involve collecting information about what a YP is doing currently, whilst they are feeling low in mood. An activity diary, or activity log, is a method of recording this, even if they might describe themselves as doing 'nothing', such as lying in bed, scrolling their phone, or sleeping. Activity monitoring in this way is often used for this intervention as a between-session home task. Reviewing the information brought back by a YP will then allow for curious conversations and the beginning of a plan to introduce a new activity.

When planning a new activity, it can be beneficial to pick things that match a YP's values, the things that matter to them. Once new activities are introduced, you will support the YP to reflect on how this impacts their mood, consider building on the activities, and plan for increasing activity further going forward in a balanced way. You can act as a supportive, 'coaching', and motivating person to the YP at this stage, reinforcing any changes made through praise and encouragement.

Box 5.3   BA case example continued

The case example of Sam is continued below, again fully anonymised and making use of a pseudonym.

After getting a clear understanding of what Sam's days and levels of activity looked like whilst they were low in mood, their EMHP was able to support them to make some behavioural changes.

Sam worked with their EMHP to add in creative activities, connect more regularly with their friends, and start going to rehearsals for a performance they wanted to take part in. These were set up as SMART goals, such as "I will do one creative activity a week", which helped make them manageable and achievable for Sam.

Sam was able to meet all of their goals by the end of the brief intervention. They reported that they felt more energised from seeing their friends and doing creative activities, compared to what they had been doing before which was staying home and being on their phone. Having considered their values as part of the intervention, Sam had re-evaluated how they were spending their time and added in activities that aligned with what mattered to them.

Sam told their practitioner that the work had helped them understand themself better. The EMHP supported Sam to think about how they could carry on with BA work after the sessions finished, continuing to increase activities that mattered to them. This also gave them a plan for what to do in the future if their mood dipped again.

Many EMHP courses around the country utilise a specific manualised approach to BA, known as Brief BA (Pass & Reynolds, 2021). This manualised approach has been clinically trialled, giving it a robust evidence base. It has been developed to include handouts for YP and parents to support each session, which are all available within a book that acts as a practitioner manual and guide. These resources make it popular with trainee and qualified EMHPs alike.

Worry Management

Where problematic worry (sometimes referred to as generalised anxiety or GAD where diagnostic criteria are met) is the identified presenting problem for a young person, you can offer WM. This intervention is behavioural in nature and can be useful for helping YP where the *act* (or behaviour) of worrying is the main thing getting in the way of day-to-day life and things the young person would rather be doing.

Charlotte Temple, a specialist lecturer on CWP, EMHP, Supervisor, SWP, and HI CBT programmes and an experienced CBT therapist, has a keen interest in WM for low-intensity practitioners (EMHPs and CWPs). Charlotte says,

> In practice WM will often be one of the most frequent interventions used by EMHPs and CWPs. The key point of the intervention is around helping YP manage the process of worrying itself, moving away from the content of worry thoughts.

This approach, managing worry as a behaviour, fits with the behavioural approach offered by EMHPs, whilst supporting YP in managing their worries in a different way. YP who are 'worriers' (and this is often the way YP who experience problematic worry have been described or would describe themselves) are often used to trying to address each individual worry as it comes along. They may do this in a variety of ways, common methods including seeking reassurance from others, preparing for things an excessive amount, making lots of very detailed plans, or simply spending a lot of time worrying about it. There is often a belief that worrying is helpful and will prevent the worst from happening.

This intervention will spend very little time on exploring the content of individual worries. It can be useful to know a little bit about what types of worries YP have as this supports implementing some of the new WM techniques, but the individual worries won't be addressed. This can be a surprise to some YP. Instead, the intervention addresses the behaviour or process of worry and supports YP to change what they do about their worries.

Box 5.4   WM case example from practice

An example of a WM case from practice has been provided by an EMHP, who will remain unnamed to preserve the anonymity of the YP they supported. The case example below is fully anonymised and makes use of a pseudonym, Lucy, which is not the YP's real name.

Lucy, age 10 years, was described by both her Mum and her class teacher as 'a worrier'. She described lots of worries about a variety of situations, with a current particular focus on school and the move up to high school at the end of the year. She would have thoughts such as "What if I don't do well?", "What if I get lost in the big building?", and "What if I don't make any friends?". Any time that there were tests in school would be particularly difficult for Lucy.

When worrying she would feel scared and sad, and described feeling 'butterflies' in her tummy, a 'shiver' down her spine, and her heart pounding in her chest. Mum shared that Lucy often seemed tense and could be very irritable with family. Lucy's teacher told the EMHP that she would struggle to concentrate in class, seeming very distracted. Lucy would ask the adults around her, at home and in school, if she would "Be ok?" or if she was "Doing well enough?" often. Lucy's attendance at school had begun to suffer due to her worries.

Supporting YP to identify the type of worry they are experiencing is one of the first steps in WM. The types of worry are generally categorised as 'real' or 'hypothetical'; however, many EMHPs choose to adjust the language here to be more child-friendly.

Amelia Bellmon is an associate lecturer on CWP and EMHP programmes, qualified as a CWP and HI CBT therapist, and an experienced low-intensity clinical supervisor. Amelia says,

> Using the world real to describe one type of worry could potentially lead a YP to think we're saying that the other type of worry, hypothetical worries, aren't real, and this could feel quite invalidating. I prefer to use the term 'problem solvable worries' instead of 'real'. I also find the word hypothetical isn't very child friendly, so I call those worries 'what if worries'. If a YP has a different way of describing them, then I'd use their own language too.

Once the YP understands the two different types of worry, they can practice sorting their worries. There are then different ways of dealing with each type of worry. If the worry is 'real' (or 'problem solvable'), then a problem-solving technique can be taught and utilised. This involves helping the YP list all the possible things that could be done in response to the problem, identify what is good and bad about each option, and then choose the best option to try out, scheduling in a time to do this and who might be needed to help them with it.

If the worry is 'hypothetical' (or a 'what if worry'), then the YP is supported to recognise this and understand that there isn't anything they can do to change whether the worry will happen or not. They can then make use of 'let it go' techniques to take their mind off the worry. You may spend time helping the YP develop their own range of 'let it go' techniques, finding out what is most helpful for them.

One final element of WM is working on tolerance of uncertainty. YP who worry tend to dislike uncertainty, in part because uncertainty can give lots of space for hypothetical or 'what if' worries to take over. Situations that are uncertain are often managed by trying to create more certainty, through preparing, asking lots of questions, or only doing certain things (avoiding those things that are very uncertain). However, the problem with this is that life is often uncertain, and absolute certainty is hard to achieve, particularly if you want to go about your life and enjoy it.

Tolerating uncertainty work involves supporting YP to change their behaviour around uncertainty (again, sticking with a behavioural approach that fits with the EMHP role), so that, instead of creating more certainty, they can get used to being ok with some uncertainty. This is done in a similar way to a graded exposure intervention (read on in this chapter for more detail on this intervention). This involves trying out easier steps towards uncertainty first and gradually getting more used to it and how it feels. Charlotte Temple (who we met earlier in the chapter) highlighted to us the effectiveness of this element and how well it can fit with a low-intensity, behaviour-based approach to WM.

Box 5.5   WM case example continued

The case example of Lucy is continued below, again fully anonymised and making use of a pseudonym.

Lucy and her EMHP worked through a WM intervention, firstly helping Lucy understand the different types of worries. Where Lucy had a 'problem-solvable' worry, her

EMHP helped her to learn techniques for what to do about it. For the "what if" (hypothetical) worries, which were most of the worries Lucy had, her EMHP helped her to learn how to let these go.

With agreement from Lucy, the EMHP shared resources with Mum and her class teacher. This helped them to know how to support Lucy when she was worrying too.

Getting used to uncertainty was a particularly helpful strategy for Lucy, with Mum commenting on what a difference it had made. When Lucy became a little bit more comfortable with not knowing exactly what would happen, or trying things that were new, Mum noticed that there were a lot less 'what if' worries and less questions from Lucy about if things would 'be ok'.

Exposure

Graded exposure can be offered for anxiety presentations where avoidance is a key factor in keeping the problem going (maintenance). Presentations appropriate for this intervention might include specific phobia, separation anxiety, symptoms of panic (subthreshold for panic disorder) or anxiety with a social element, and related avoidance behaviours (not meeting diagnostic criteria for social phobia).

Graded exposure is based on supporting the YP to have gradually increasing amounts of contact with the object or situation causing anxiety.

Box 5.6   Exposure case example from practice

An example of an exposure case from practice has been provided by an EMHP, who will remain unnamed to preserve the anonymity of the YP they supported. The case example below is fully anonymised and makes use of a pseudonym, Jayden, which is not the YP's real name.

> Jayden, age 9 years, had a fear of dogs that was caus-
> ing a significant problem for him and his family. There
> was no identifiable trigger for Jayden's fear, but he strongly
> expressed his thoughts that "dogs are horrible" and "a dog
> will bite me". The thought of being around a dog made
> Jayden scared, and he described his heart beating 'really
> fast'. He would sometimes get angry if his Mum tried to get
> him to play out or go to the shop with her, for fear of seeing
> a dog.
>
> Jayden found it very difficult to go to places that might
> have dogs around, meaning that his family had to think
> carefully about where they went. Jayden would no longer
> go over to friend's houses for tea or sleepovers and would
> only play in his own yard, much preferring to stay at home
> to 'feel safe'. Jayden would insist on having a lift to school
> rather than walking, again due to the fear of seeing a dog.

Having identified the YP's anxiety-inducing object (e.g., dog)
or situation (e.g., speaking to someone they don't know), you will
support YP to build a list of examples of related things that would
make them feel anxious. These can then be rated and ordered, so
that the result is a list from the least anxiety-provoking example to
the most anxiety-provoking example. Rating can be done using a
number, from 0 to 10, or a percentage, from 0 to 100%.

Where possible, there should be enough things on the list to
gradually work up, without too big a jump in the level of anxiety. For example, if YP has a dog phobia, watching a video of a
dog jumping and barking might create anxiety that YP rates as
three out of ten. However, walking across a field where dogs are
running around off the lead might create anxiety rated as ten out
of ten. This is obviously a large jump, so it would be helpful for
you to support YP to fill in the gaps. Finding other examples of
things that give some anxiety, at ratings in between three and ten,
helps ensure that the exposure is graded and more likely to be
successful.

The content of exposure sessions would include supporting the YP to have contact with things from their list. Lists are
sometimes drawn out as steps or ladders, with the term for this

being a hierarchy. To get the best outcome from exposure, you will support YP to really focus on the task, without using distractions or avoidance techniques (such as thinking of something else or not looking directly at the object).

To give an example of a situation-based exposure intervention (rather than object-based), a YP might be supported to manage their anxiety over speaking to people they don't know. Their ladder might include lower-level steps such as paying for something in a shop where they have to say 'thank you' to the cashier, or asking for a ticket on a bus, through to higher level steps such as going to a social event with people they are less familiar with, or speaking to a new person at school or college.

Across sessions, you will help the YP work their way up the ladder, gradually getting used to contact with the object or situation causing them anxiety and developing new learning that they can manage it and will be ok.

Within this intervention, it is fully acknowledged that doing exposure steps and encountering something that makes you anxious isn't always easy – we wanted to be clear that we recognise this! Therefore, it is even more important to make the steps manageable and start with things that are low level, to support YP to experience success early on and be able to build on this as steps become trickier. Having an end goal in sight and ensuring YP is on board with wanting things to be different also helps.

Parent-Led Anxiety

As an EMHP, you are trained not only to work with YP directly but also to offer support via parents or carers. For clarity of writing purposes, we will continue this section using the term 'parent'; however, we would like to make clear that any adult who has regular and primary care responsibility for a child can be appropriate for this support. This might include, but is not limited to, birth, step, or adoptive parents, grandparents or other adult family members with a direct care responsibility for the child, foster carers, kinship carers, and more.

This type of support is sometimes referred to as 'parenting work', or parent-led CBT. There is strong evidence to demonstrate that working via parents is effective, particularly with children of primary school age.

Nicky Nolan is a trainee EMHP and particularly enjoys the parent-led work and interactions with parents. She tells us, "Working this way can have a real impact on making changes at home, supporting longer lasting change for YP".

This work to support parents is obviously a distinct difference to the PWP or MHWP role. EMHPs and CWPs will often spend considerable time interacting with parents, carers, and other adults in the systems supporting children and YP.

For children of primary age presenting with anxiety difficulties, including generalised anxiety, separation anxiety, or phobias, you are taught to deliver a parent-led CBT-informed approach supported by a book, *Helping Your Child with Fears and Worries* (Creswell & Willetts, 2019), which parents work through alongside support.

The approach, which has been clinically trialled for effectiveness, is designed as a combination of face-to-face and telephone-based support. This can improve access for parents who may have other responsibilities and competing demands on their time. Support is delivered directly to the parent, or parents, with the child generally not attending the sessions. The only exception to this is the assessment session, where it can be beneficial to meet the child and ensure their voice is included in gathering information on the problem.

The intervention itself is based around taking a stepped, or graded, method to challenging fear and worry and supporting parents to develop a 'have a go' approach alongside their child. The underpinning theory is exposure and inhibitory learning, which means supporting the child or young person to "have a go" and encounter the thing that they would usually avoid due to anxiety, so that they can learn that the outcome they are afraid of doesn't usually happen, or if it does – they can cope with it!

Parent-Led Behaviour

A second intervention delivered directly to a parent or carer is the parent-led intervention for low-level problems with behaviour. This intervention is designed to support parents and carers of children aged 10 years and under and, as with the previously described parent-led intervention, has strong evidence for its effectiveness.

Gareth Edwards is a specialist lecturer on CWP and EMHP programmes, a CBT therapist, and is experienced in supporting parents and families. Gareth acknowledges that talking about parenting can be emotive and tells us, "It is not uncommon for practitioners to feel that they are insensitively or clumsily prying when completing an assessment and gathering information about the problem". He shares that holding onto the core competencies of practice, such as curiosity and collaboration, while consistently giving clarity on the practitioner's role and remit, and why you are asking the questions you are, can help manage this.

The intervention is designed to support parents of children, between 2 and 9 years old, presenting with mild problems with their behaviour. These problems should not meet clinical thresholds or criteria for diagnosable disorders, such as Conduct Disorder, defined within *The Diagnostic and Statistical Manual of Mental Disorders, Fifth Edition* (APA, 2013).

The intervention emphasises broad principles of parenting and enhances parenting strategies, rather than prescribing specific techniques. It aims to prevent escalation of problem behaviours, meaning that it is a preventative intervention in fitting with the remit of EMHPs. Gathering information on specific problem behaviours at assessment stage is important and can be effectively done by use of curious questioning and exploring a recent incident (via RIA). As with all PP work, parents are supported to set goals to work towards, identifying what they would like to be different and what they would hope to achieve via support.

The intervention is split into two broad sections, with the first focusing on promoting and enhancing the parent-child relationship and the second including routines, boundaries, and limit setting. Across the early sessions, you will support the parent to understand their child's current behaviour and what might impact on this, in fitting with CBT-informed approaches and psychoeducation.

You will then support the parent to introduce time for focused play with their child, sometimes referred to as 'special time', with emphasis on this being child-led. A nice metaphor that can be used to explain the rationale for this can be that of putting money into a piggy bank to invest. In a similar way, spending positive time together is explained as investing in the relationship and their child.

Following this, you will work with the parent on making use of more regular and specific praise with their child. Research shows that where children are praised in a way that is specific, such as "you've really taken your time with that picture, well done", as opposed to more generic or outcome-focused, such as "you're excellent at drawing", it can increase motivation and positively influence self-esteem and self-evaluation.

The later sessions include supporting the parent to manage unwanted behaviours through strategies such as improving boundaries and expectations, giving effective commands, withdrawing attention (i.e., not responding) when unwanted behaviours are displayed, using calm time, and enforcing consequences when boundaries are crossed.

It is important to clarify that, within strategies for enforcing consequences, there is strong emphasis on promoting non-violent and non-punitive discipline approaches. It is also important to be clear that withdrawing attention may not be possible if a child is behaving in a way that is dangerous or destructive. In these instances, the use of calm time and/or consequences may be unavoidable, so this is discussed with parents and planned for.

One of the key methods utilised in parent-led interventions, with strong evidence for its effectiveness, is brought in here. Modelling and rehearsal are experiential learning methods that support parents to 'have a go' and practice skills and strategies before going home to try them with their child. This means, in a general sense, that you and the parent practice (sometimes called 'role play', but we acknowledge this word can put people off) within the session, one person 'being' the child and one 'being' the parent.

At some points, the parent might be best placed to be the child, so they can give examples of what their child might say, and you will 'be' the parent, so you can demonstrate (model) new strategies and ways of responding. At other points, you might take on the role of the child, so that the parent can 'be' themself and practice different strategies and responses.

Gareth Edwards (who we met earlier) highlights the benefits of collaboration and teamwork in parent interventions. He acknowledges,

Many parents may begin the process somewhat pessimistically, due to their view of what the problem is and/or previous experiences of working with services. However, parents' knowledge, experience of their child, and insight, coupled with the practitioner's approaches, and an effective therapeutic relationship, can produce a really successful intervention and outcome.

Qualifications

EMHP training is awarded the qualification of a Postgraduate Diploma or Graduate Diploma, with 120 credits to be completed, generally split across six modules.

Modules are defined in the curriculum as follows:

Module 1: Children and young people's MH settings: context and values

Module 2: Assessment and engagement

Module 3: Evidence-based interventions for common MH problems with children and YP (theory and skills)

Module 4: Working, assessing, and engaging in education settings

Module 5: Common problems and processes in education settings

Module 6: Interventions for emerging MH difficulties in education settings

It should be noted that these are the modules as defined in the national curriculum, but there may be differences in naming and module breakdown across different higher education institutes or training providers. More detailed discussion of the qualifications can be found in Chapter 8 – Being a Trainee.

Education Specialist Role and Whole School Approaches

As mentioned earlier, a key element of the EMHP role, distinct from direct 1:1 work with children, YP, or parents and carers, is that of supporting WSAs to MH and wellbeing. It should be noted that the term WSA is commonly used, but this can also be adjusted to Whole College Approaches where that is more appropriate.

WSAs are supported by eight guiding principles, as outlined in the HM Government and Children and Young People's Mental Health Coalition document 'Promoting children and young people's mental health and wellbeing: a whole school or college approach'. These eight principles are as follows:

- Leadership and management
- Ethos and environment
- Curriculum, teaching, and learning
- Student voice
- Staff development, health, and wellbeing
- Identifying need and monitoring impact
- Working with parents, families, and carers
- Targeted support and appropriate referrals

These principles were developed based upon evidence as well as practitioner feedback about what works and building on what many schools and colleges are already doing across the country.

WSA, in practice, can include a range of activities for EMHPs, including, but not limited to, conducting audits on school MH and wellbeing provision and need, providing workshops and assemblies that are universal (for all) in nature, providing workshops and groupwork that are targeted (for identified YP), engaging and supporting staff understanding of MH, and consulting with staff.

Ally Boyne, a specialist lecturer and marking coordinator on EMHP and CWP programmes, and a CBT therapist, is passionate about WSA. She says,

> WSA are integral to the EMHP role but sometimes fall under the radar during the training year when the focus is often on building skills in assessment and intervention. However, it plays such a key role in prevention of MH difficulties and promotion of good MH and wellbeing, that putting time into prioritising and embedding this into the MHST offer can make a significant difference. We should champion WSA as EMHPs!

Conclusion

We hope that this chapter has given you a good insight into the EMHP role and what this can look like in practice. Is this the PP role for you? If not, please revisit Chapter 2 or 3 to learn about the adult roles of PWP and MHWP or Chapter 4 to explore the CWP role.

If the EMHP role does sound like a good fit, then that's wonderful and welcome to the MHST – you may want to move on to Chapter 6 and beyond to continue exploring your career options.

Box 5.7 References and wider reading

American Psychiatric Association. (2013). *The diagnostic and statistical manual of mental disorders. 5th Edition.* American Psychiatric Association.

Anna Freud Centre. (2020). *Mentally healthy schools: Whole-school approach.* https://www.mentallyhealthyschools.org.uk/whole-school-approach/

Creswell, C., & Willetts, L. (2019). *Helping your child with fears and worries. 2nd Edition.* Robinson.

Department of Health & NHS England. (2015). *Future in mind: Promoting, protecting, and improving our children and young people's mental health and wellbeing.*

HM Government. (2011). *No health without mental health: A cross-government mental health outcomes strategy for people of all ages.*

Mental Health Taskforce. (2014). *Five year forward view.*

Pass, L., & Reynolds, S. (2021). *Brief behavioural activation for adolescent depression: A clinician's manual and session-by-session guide.* Jessica Kingsley Publishers.

Wolpert, M., Harris, R., Hodges, S., Fuggle, P., James, R., & Wiener, A. (2019). *THRIVE framework for system change.* CAMHS Press.

Chapter 6

Routes into the Profession

Introduction

Psychological practitioner (PP) training courses are completed as part of an employed role. This means that you cannot apply directly or solely to the training provider (which is usually a university) to be able to train as a PP. Instead, you must find a job and begin employment as a trainee Psychological Wellbeing Practitioner (PWP), Mental Health Wellbeing Practitioner (MHWP), Children's Wellbeing Practitioner (CWP), or Education Mental Health Practitioner (EMHP), or an apprenticeship position as a PWP, to undertake the training.

Courses generally take 12 months to complete under a training contract. On completion of the course, the aim is that services will continue the employment for the practitioner under a qualified contract, with the corresponding increase in salary.

But how do you get a training role in the first place? Where should you look if you're interested in training as a PP?

A good place to begin is the National Health Service (NHS) jobs website, as most PP training roles are employed via the NHS. Searching for the titles of the roles and the word "trainee" will most likely bring up any available opportunities, with the opportunity to filter results based on the area you wish to work in. There are a range of training providers offering PP courses in all regions of England, with roles available alongside these.

As well as the NHS, some PP trainee roles are offered via other types of organisations, such as mental health charities. These may form part of local mental health partnership offers. This means that knowing the types of mental health service providers and local

DOI: 10.4324/9781003542049-6

offers in the area you wish to train and work can also give you additional places to look for advertised roles. Organisations may advertise available roles and training opportunities via their own websites, via any social media platforms they use, or via more generalised job websites. As with the NHS jobs website, searching for words and terms related to the job titles, plus the word 'trainee', can bring up appropriate results.

Once you find an advertisement for a trainee PP role, what do you need to consider next? Because these roles incorporate the training course alongside employment, it is important to consider the academic level of training when selecting trainee roles to apply for. This is so you can check you have the required qualifications and experience for entry onto the training course.

Training for PP roles is offered at the following levels:

- Undergraduate level, a level 6 qualification resulting in the award of Graduate Certificate or Graduate Diploma
- Postgraduate level, a level 7 qualification resulting in the award of Postgraduate Certificate or Postgraduate Diploma
- Apprenticeship level, a level 6 qualification, however only currently offered for the PWP role

The awarded qualifications for undergraduate and postgraduate level study tend to be a certificate for PWPs and MHWPs and a diploma for CWPs and EMHPs. This is based upon the number of modules completed and credits awarded, with 60 credits (usually three modules) being required for a certificate and 120 credits (usually six modules) for a diploma.

More detail on training is included further on in this book (see Chapter 8 – Being a Trainee). However, specific requirements for training programmes would need to be acquired from the training provider or checked in the details of the specific trainee role job advertisement.

We would recommend checking information about the training provider, or higher education institute (HEI), that offers the training element of the role. Universities or training providers will usually have websites giving information about courses, about their locations and sites, and often information on student services and even student experience.

You might want to consider where the training provider is based geographically, as they are not necessarily going to be in the same area as your employing organisation. For example, CWPs who train in the North West will train via the Psychological Therapies Training Centre in Prestwich, near Manchester. This is currently the only training provider offering the CWP course in the North West. Therefore, trainee CWPs based anywhere across the region will be required to travel to this provider for their teaching days. This may not be far for trainees based in Manchester, Bury, or Rochdale, but a much longer commute for trainees based in Chester, on the Wirral, or in Blackpool, for example. This may need considering, particularly if you are not a driver, although there are often groups of trainees travelling in to teaching together, and car-sharing may be a possibility. It may also be that venues for teaching have good public transport links available.

It may sound obvious, but it is also useful to spend some time thinking more specifically about which of the PP roles appeals most before you look for training positions or begin to apply. Although there are broad similarities between the roles, all supporting people via the use of evidence-based, cognitive behavioural therapy (CBT)-informed, low-intensity interventions, there are also key differences. The training courses are not interchangeable, and, once trained, you need to register and work in your specified role (see Chapter 9 – Professional Ethics for more information on registration).

Reading through the role-specific chapters of this book (see Chapter 2 – Being a PWP, Chapter 3 – Being an MHWP, Chapter 4 – Being a CWP, and Chapter 5 – Being an EMHP) will give you a clearer idea of the specifics of each role. You might want to consider if you'd rather work with adult clients or with children, young people (YP), and families, as well as considering the setting you'd like to work in. For example, would you want to work in a specific low-intensity or Step 2 service as a PWP, alongside a Community Mental Health Team or setting accessed by clients with more severe mental health difficulties as an MHWP, in a community or primary care setting as a CWP, or in an education setting such as a school or college as an EMHP.

Marianne Tay, a course lead for an MHWP programme and an experienced CBT therapist, emphasises this need to consider specifically which of the PP roles is right for you when you begin to apply for a job as a trainee. Marianne tells us, in relation to recruiting for trainee MHWPs,

> We look for the reasons that the individual wants to be an MHWP specifically, as opposed to another PP role. We want to make sure trainees are passionate about community mental healthcare and want to work with adult clients experiencing severe mental health difficulties, not just mental health in general.

Backgrounds

We know that many who train to be PPs may come from a background of having studied psychology in some form previously, be this at A-level, undergraduate, or master's level. Having some previous experience and understanding of psychology can lead people to want to train in roles where they can put this into use in their daily work, which is certainly the case as a PWP, MHWP, CWP, or EMHP.

However, a background in psychology is not necessarily a pre-requisite to becoming a PP. There are a wide range of backgrounds, in terms of education, previous training, previous employment, and more broadly life experiences, that can lead people to want to train and work as PPs.

Laura Spence, a qualified CWP, recognises this, telling us, "One of the many positive qualities to this training is that it can upskill professionals who may not have originally chosen a career in psychology".

Kirsten Brown is a qualified MHWP and also appreciates this, saying

> I am a big fan of the fact that with the MHWP role there is less of an emphasis on academic achievements in the sense of paid courses, and more of an emphasis on merit, such as people who have worked in fields related to mental health and have gained proven experience. I believe this is an excellent opportunity to work in mental health, that does not exclude those who may have relevant experiences.

I (Kirsty, one of your authors) did not study psychology at A-level or undergraduate level. With a BA in Screen Studies and Imaginative Writing (who would have thought that the writing element would end up coming in handy…) and three years working at an American summer camp with adults and children with disabilities, I ended up somewhat by chance in the healthcare field. Initially working as a support worker in an adult mental health unit, I then realised that work with YP was more appealing for me. I worked as a support worker on a CYPMHS inpatient unit, during which time I gained valuable experience and had the opportunity to complete a counselling skills course and a BSc in Behaviour Analysis and Intervention. This meant that, when I saw an advertisement for a trainee role on the pilot cohort of the CWP training, it seemed like the obvious next step for me. This was my circuitous route to the role I am now so passionate about.

It may also be that you are coming to PP training from a background of experience and without an undergraduate degree. As noted in the introduction to training in the section above, this is also a valid route. There are options to complete PWP, CWP, EMHP, and MHWP courses as graduate certificates or diplomas (as opposed to postgraduate certificates or diplomas).

Matthew Beaton, a principal mental health practitioner and honorary lecturer on an MHWP programme, backs this up, telling us "A degree is not always required. Many training providers offer undergraduate routes".

Matthew also points out that some may have a degree but in an entirely unrelated field, and this is also ok. He says, "If you do have a degree in a non-psychology related field it won't negatively impact your application".

Others may come to the roles from working within wider mental health or wellbeing settings and seeing the PP roles in action. Matthew Draper, a current trainee CWP, had previously been an assistant practitioner in a CAMHS team, working alongside qualified and trainee CWPs. Matthew tells us,

> I was able to shadow the qualified practitioner and took a lot of learning from seeing their practice. My team leader spoke to me and asked if this role was something I would look to apply for as a progression route.

It can also be common for those with lived (which generally refers to historic) experience and/or living (referring to current or ongoing) experience of accessing support for their mental health, either their own experience or via a family member or friend, to be inspired to work in the field of mental health. It is widely understood, and backed up by research, that there can be a range of benefits and values to this lived and living experience in enhancing the work of trained mental health professionals, and this is no different within the PP roles.

Matthew Beaton (the first Matthew we heard from ... getting confusing yet?) tells us, "Applications from individuals with lived experience of mental health difficulties, who have developed effective coping and self-management strategies, are warmly welcomed".

What is important to also note, however, is the need for any trainee (or indeed qualified) PP to consider their own wellbeing. When undertaking training, it is important to recognise the demands of this and ensure that it is something you feel ready to undertake.

Karen Rea, a PWP Programme Lead, tells us, "A trainee PWP needs to be emotionally and psychologically resilient for what is a very interesting but challenging training year".

Marianne Tay (who we met earlier in the chapter) says,

> Make sure this is the right decision for you at the right time. Training as an MHWP is a fantastic opportunity and propels you right into the heart of mental health treatment in the UK. However, it is demanding. Whilst it is some of the most rewarding work you can do, it is inevitable that you will be exposed to some sensitive and potentially distressing topics including trauma and abuse. You need to ensure that you are at a point in your own career and where relevant, recovery journey, to support others without harming your own wellbeing.

Whilst Marianne's advice is most relevant to the MHWP role, specifically working with those with more severe mental health difficulties, it is still relevant to consider with any PP role. In the roles working at early intervention and the first point of contact with mental health services, end of the spectrum (e.g., PWP, CWP, and EMHP), there is still always the chance that someone will disclose to you something that is potentially upsetting.

It is always beneficial for applicants to any of the PP roles to have some experience of working with mental health. This does not have to be employment in a paid role and can include unpaid or voluntary positions or experience gained as an additional aspect of a substantive (main) job role. Some training programmes include this experience of work with mental health as an essential criterion (more about essential and desirable criteria is included later in the chapter).

Marianne backs this up, telling us,

> We really value trainees who have experience working in a mental health setting, as this reassures us that they are not going to be intimidated or overwhelmed by clients, and that they can communicate with people in distress. The work experience does not need to be extensive. It could be volunteering for Samaritans, SHOUT or another mental health charity, alongside a main job or a training course.

Sara Yunus is a service lead for a Mental Health Support Team, where EMHPs are based, and has also been part of the tutor team for a PP training course. Sara notes that when recruiting trainees for the CYP roles (EMHP or CWP), she would be looking for candidates who specifically have experience of working with children, YP, and families. This does not have to be in a mental health setting but demonstrating that you have worked with CYP in some way is important. Sara adds, "If you can talk about this experience in a positive way and with enthusiasm, that's a bonus".

Widening Access

It is generally acknowledged that there is an ongoing need to recruit, train, and, importantly, retain a diverse workforce of psychological professionals that can be reflective of the communities served. The PP workforce and the cohorts of trainees on PP training programmes each year tend to be predominantly white and predominantly female. There is an acknowledged need to increase representation within the workforce for certain sociodemographic groups, with the aim behind this being to increase engagement and uptake of support for those communities and populations.

For example, increasing recruitment of men in the PP roles may support more men, across the age range and potentially also men from minoritised ethnic backgrounds, to seek support for anxiety or depression. This is important, as we know from research that men are less likely to talk about their mental health and access professional support due to gender-based stigma.

Safa Asif, a qualified CWP, tells us that increasing representation was a key factor in their desire to train as a PP. Safa says,

> Being Muslim, from a South Asian background, and having experienced mental health issues in my family, I wanted to ensure YP from different ethnic backgrounds, had someone they could relate too. There are not many people of colour within the mental health field. Increased representation is much needed as we know that those from minoritised ethnic communities are at higher risk of developing mental health issues. There can be massive stigma within different cultures and communities, and I wanted to make sure I could tap into this and create that awareness and understanding. Minoritised communities can often be labelled as 'hard to reach' but in fact we, as mental health services, are hard for them to reach.

Safa goes on to tell us about how their own culture influences their work as a CWP. She tells us,

> I bring in my own experiences and culture to help me ensure that culture and race are discussed in all aspects of our work. I do sometimes feel that, if I don't say it, would another person who is White British mention this? Ensuring we are all comfortable in asking questions and being curious when working with YP from a different background to ourselves, is key. Some may feel awkward about it initially, which I understand but we need to start getting comfortable with being uncomfortable. This is how we grow. It has been going on for too long now and the system needs to change. I hope that I am part of that positive change.

If you are reading this book as a hopeful future PP from a minoritised community or background, we would encourage you to keep considering this as a career pathway. This is not to ignore the well-documented structural and systemic barriers for some to accessing the required experiences, training, or opportunities that might lead to a PP training role. These barriers and inequalities are very real, and in writing this book, both authors recognise our own areas of privilege, in particular as white women in this field.

Widening Access and Participation initiatives in the NHS are designed to support a commitment to putting in place a health care workforce that is representative of the communities it serves. Further information on these initiatives can be found via national and local NHS sources.

Applying for Trainee Roles

This section will include general advice for applying for a trainee PP role, as well as drawing on those who employ and train PPs to hear what they might look for and want to see in applications or interviews for trainee posts. However, because there are variations in processes across the PP roles and between different HEIs, education providers, and employing organisations, our advice will remain broad and general rather than specific.

Some of this advice and information may also be useful to consider at points further into a career as a PP, which is also covered in Chapter 10 (Mastering the Job Market), albeit without the focus on the training year and trainee positions.

The first advice that can be given in relation to reviewing job advertisements and completing application forms is to ensure that you read everything through thoroughly. Even read things through a couple of times, to ensure that you are clear on what they are looking for, and on what criteria are essential or desirable for the post. When looking for a trainee position, it is also particularly important to ensure that the training element is included in the title of the role and job description, to make sure that it is not a role where they expect you to already be qualified!

The required criteria for candidates to meet are usually included in the job description, or sometimes within an additional document called a person specification. The criteria might be split into lists of essential or desirable criteria or listed within a table with columns that indicate along the side whether each criterion is essential or desirable.

These columns may also indicate where the employer expects you to demonstrate that you can meet these criteria, for example, via the application form, via references, via document or certificate checks, or via interview. This is useful to consider so that you can make the best use of the application to demonstrate your skills and have an idea of which elements you will be asked to demonstrate via the questions in an interview.

We want to acknowledge that it can be daunting to begin filling in an application form, particularly if you've not done many before. Where possible, give yourself plenty of time to work on this. However, keep in mind that some job advertisements are closed to further applications once a specified number have been received. With PP trainee positions being in high demand, it may be that application numbers and limits are reached quickly, even within a day or two.

When completing the application form, it is important to make sure to identify how you meet all the essential criteria. Some of these may be covered by the details you are required to fill in, such as your qualifications, previous employment, and so on. Other essential criteria might need to be included in a personal statement, explaining how you meet them. For example, if you are asked to demonstrate an ability to develop good relationships with those you support, then this would be necessary to expand on in a personal or supporting statement.

It is also important to include information on how you meet as many of the desirable criteria as you can. Trainee PP posts often receive high numbers of applicants, as these funded training positions are in demand, so ensuring that you show how you can meet these additional desirable qualities and skills will give you a better chance of being shortlisted to make it to the interview stage.

This final advice may sound obvious but is likely still worth saying. Checking spelling is important, so that your application looks as professional as possible. If the application system you are using is online and doesn't have the spellcheck facility included, it can be useful to write out any supporting statements (or longer blocks of text) in a Word document first so that you can spell check it there. You can then usually copy and paste this back into the online form.

Getting someone else to read through your application and any required supporting statement can also spot spelling mistakes and check that it reads clearly and coherently. It doesn't necessarily matter if the person reading it for you is knowledgeable about the roles, or this field of work, as the focus of reading through is about checking how clear it is. They may also be able to check against the essential and desirable criteria for you, to ensure that you have mentioned how you meet them.

Interviews

Interviews for PP training posts may be conducted in different ways by different employing organisations and education providers. Some may run one interview, with representatives of both the employing organisation and the training provider on the panel. Others may have separate interviews.

With changes in modes of working over recent years, there may be some interviews conducted remotely, via an online platform. This can involve a different skill set than managing a face-to-face interview, so it may be worth practicing using online platforms or getting someone to call you to practice ahead of the interview if you are less familiar with this.

It is important to remember to be punctual for your interview, be this turning up on time at a location or joining an online meeting promptly, to give a good first impression. If travelling somewhere in person, check your route and any public transport or parking requirements as needed. If joining an interview remotely, make sure that you have the right link or code to hand in plenty of time.

Although PP roles can involve working in community settings, or with children and YP, which may require adopting a less formal approach to support engagement, it is important to remember to convey professionalism during the interview and associated interactions. Professionalism can be demonstrated through choice of clothing, manner, language, and wider communication (verbal, non-verbal, and written), as well as via the content you refer to. Although interviewers will want to get a sense of your personality as an individual, they will be looking for someone who can represent their organisation well during the training year (both in practice and when on training days) and beyond.

However conducted, interviews will all be geared towards identifying your suitability for the role (e.g., are you someone with the right skills, knowledge, and attributes to make a good PP) and for the training (e.g., do you have the right qualifications and/or ability to study at the level required, to complete the qualification within the training year?).

Many interview panels and processes now include those with lived experience of accessing mental health support. These may be individuals who have accessed support in the past via the organisation and are now part of a participation or lived experience panel. If you are applying for one of the roles working with YP (CWP or EMHP), then the lived experience representative may be a child or YP, or a parent or carer of someone who has been supported.

This inclusion of lived experience within recruitment is very much in line with the ethos and principles of the NHS Talking Therapies for Anxiety and Depression (formerly Improving Access to Psychological Therapies) and Children and YP's Psychological Trainings (CYP PT – formerly Children and YP's Improving Access to Psychological Therapies) programmes. Within CYP PT, this also links into the principle of 'participation' (see Chapters 4 and 5, on being a CWP or EMHP for further details of these principles) and is included as one of the nine participation priorities, priority number 5 being 'involve YP in recruitment'.

When you are being interviewed for a potential training place on a PP course, what are the interview panel looking for?

Paul Thompson is a qualified PWP, senior lecturer in Mental Health, and Director of the Psychological Professionals' Development Hub. From his experience recruiting to PWP training courses, he says,

> Interviewers are looking for applicants who understand a bit about what the PWP role involves, not just in theory but in practice too. They want to see that you know about what guided self-help is, that you have some knowledge of CBT interventions, stepped care, and that you understand the importance of managing risk and caseloads.

Paul adds, "Interviewers don't expect you to know *everything* about the role – that is why you're interviewing for a training role after all – but they do expect you to have done some research".

Karen Rea (who we met earlier in the chapter) tells us that

Successful applicants that are appointed to training have demonstrated that they have a good understanding of the role and the work that PPs do. The programme focuses on the development of CBT based skills through evidence based clinical practice as well as academic achievement and potential trainees need to be aware of this requirement and enter training by committing to engaging in this process from commencement and throughout their career.

Sara Yunus (who we met earlier in the chapter) is regularly involved in recruiting candidates for trainee PP posts with children and YP. She backs up what Karen has said, telling us,

We like to hear from candidates who have a clear idea of why this role and course is right for them, and why it's right for them *now*. Showing they have thought about this demonstrates a commitment to the process, and that they have checked out some information about the role.

Matthew Beaton (who we met earlier in the chapter) adds that it can also be good to highlight specifically why you are applying to that particular education provider or placement organisation. What stood out about them to you?

Whilst Karen is talking more specifically about PWP training, Matthew brings an MHWP perspective, and Sara is referring to roles with children and YP, their advice can all be applied to any trainee PP roles.

It is always a good idea to investigate the role ahead of completing your application and certainly ahead of going for an interview. Demonstrating you understand a bit about what the role looks like, what type of work you might be doing, and what your training year might include is likely to impress the panel.

Good ways to find out some of this information might include reading up online, joining forums and groups about the roles, or speaking to someone currently training for or doing the role itself.

If you can find out specifically what the role looks like in the service you're applying to, even better. Although these roles are nationally developed, there may be some local variations and slightly different ways they are being implemented in different areas, in line with local needs, priorities, and transformation plans. Sara adds, "You can contact the service ahead of an interview and ask questions. You can even ask to visit the team in person".

And, of course, reading this book to find out more about the role will help you prepare for the interview too.

When you get to the interview stage and are preparing to answer questions from the panel, a good piece of advice is to try and share real-life examples of your skills, for every question where possible (and appropriate). There will likely be scenario-based questions, where you are asked to explain what you might do in the given situation (usually imagining you are a PP or trainee), based on your knowledge, skills, and understanding.

Marianne Tay (MHWP Course Lead, from earlier in this chapter) says,

> Many of the questions in an interview are scenario based, i.e., "what would you do if..." and the best answers are the applicants who can give an example of a time that they did this. That is one reason why it is also helpful to have some work experience that you can draw ideas from. The interview is all about demonstrating what you say you can do, and in every answer, you should give the panel an explanation of when you have previously evidenced your abilities. Remember, it is far better to be talking too much in an interview than too little! Do not assume that your application and CV will speak for themselves, you need to be able to communicate what you can do.

Sara Yunus (who we met earlier) also backs this up, telling us, "It is good to offer examples of work you have completed and show that you meet the competencies needed in the role".

Paul Thompson (who we met earlier in this chapter), whilst agreeing with the value of direct experience in mental health, also reminds us that "Transferable skills from non-clinical roles like customer service, teaching, support work and more, can help you to develop empathy, communication, and boundary-setting, so make sure you tell the interviewers about this too".

Paul continues to share from his experience, telling us,

> What really stands out in an interview is authenticity and self-awareness. Interviewers remember candidates who are clear about why they want to become a PWP and who can reflect honestly on their experiences. It is particularly impressive when someone can link their values to the ethos of the role, speak confidently about working with diverse groups, and explain how they manage stress or emotionally demanding situations. Evidence of reflective practice, for example, describing a challenging situation with a client and what you learned from it, always adds weight, and shows that you are taking meaning from your experiences.

Melissa Street, a Consultant Psychological Therapist and former CWP Programme Lead, tells us,

> Different types of experience and life skills, ability to work individually with people, and direct experience of working with YP are all of value. Try not to worry about where you've started from in your career, if it feels like your background is different or a less traditional route into psychological working. Think about how you've developed and gained experience, and where possible make links from this to what is being asked for in the PP job role. That will stand out to interviewers and recruiters.

Considering all the tips and advice included, from a range of experienced individuals, this chapter will hopefully put you in a good position to seek out your PP training role. We wish you the best of luck with the process!

Box 6.1 References and wider reading

Health Education England. (2023). *Module aims and content of education mental health practitioner for children and young people curriculum (EMHP)*. Health Education England.

Health Education England. (2023). *Module aims and content of wellbeing practitioner for children and young people curriculum (CWP). V.3.* Health Education England.

NHS England. (2023). *National curriculum for psychological wellbeing practitioner (PWP) programmes. V.4.3.* NHS England.

NHS England. (2023). *National curriculum for mental health and wellbeing practitioners.* NHS England.

NHS Jobs website – www.jobs.nhs.uk

Chapter 7

Transferable Skills

Introduction

As covered in Chapters 2–5, each psychological practitioner (PP) role has its own unique curriculum and training programme; however, each individual also brings their own set of skills to the role – transferable skills.

This chapter will cover two elements in relation to transferable skills – those which may be brought to the role by potential candidates and those which will be developed through the training and role itself.

Having noted the range of backgrounds that PPs may come from in Chapter 6, this chapter will explore the transferable skills they may bring to the training and the role. Within our understanding of transferable skills, we will not only consider those that have practical application (e.g., teachers' abilities to engage and convey ideas) but also consider the wider perspective of what a suitable candidate may bring to the role through an equality, diversity, and inclusion lens (e.g., cultural awareness of community values and needs from candidates who are representative of those communities).

There will be consideration of which skills or qualities might be deemed essential and those which are desirable, which will be particularly useful for aspiring candidates at the application or interview stage, but also for consideration within roles.

There will also be consideration of the transferable skills developed over the course of training. This may include skill in clinical record keeping, active listening, and time management,

DOI: 10.4324/9781003542049-7

Table 7.1 Opportunity to reflect on your transferable skills

Transferable Skill	Developed by

for example, which can be utilised within the role and/or future career development in health care.

Before continuing with this chapter, take a moment to consider this now: what skills do you already possess that will aid you as a PP? How have you developed these? Table 7.1 offers you a space to record your thoughts.

How Can We Identify Our Transferable Skills

To support the identification of skills, we need to reflect on our development and experiences. You may already have a good understanding of the ways in which you learn and the transferable skills you have developed over time; however, if you struggle to identify your transferable skills or you want to reflect more deeply, there are many ways to support you to do this.

It is important to consider how we learn; Erika Anderson speaks of 'learning to learn' and identifies four personal attributes, detailed in the Table 7.2. Reflection on these attributes might act as a starting point to support you on your PP journey. A journey

Table 7.2 The four attributes of 'learning to learn' and questions to reflect on in relation to these

Personal Attribute		Questions for Consideration
Aspiration	This is a desire to understand and master new skills. The idea is that by focusing on potential benefits rather than the challenge, you can increase your motivation.	What is you aspiration? What will be the benefits of you training as a PP – To yourself? To others?
Self-awareness	Through observing and reflecting on yourself, you can identify areas for development and improvement.	What reflective models do you use? What are your areas for development? What do you want to improve upon?
Curiosity	The act of asking the curious question helps you to try until you do and to think until you understand.	Cultivating curiosity in yourself and your practice. Considering the why?
Vulnerability	It is important as a PP to be compassionate to yourself. There is learning to be gained in tolerating our own mistakes. We should expect early mistakes and always endeavour to learn from them.	How do you show up as your authentic self? How does it feel? What is the impact? How do you learn from your mistakes?

that at times can be challenging, but having a sense of self-discovery, aided by becoming an effective learner, should help you navigate potential challenges. It is also an important consideration, as highlighted throughout this book, that continuous learning and development is a theme throughout your PP journey, continuing well into qualification.

Another model that may aid you in reflecting on yourself was developed by Virginia Satir, the Personal Iceberg Metaphor Model. This model asks you to consider your skills, knowledge, social role, self-image, traits, and motives.

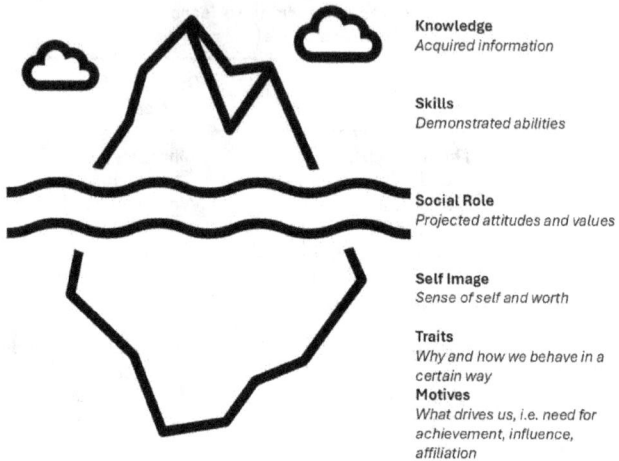

Knowledge
Acquired information

Skills
Demonstrated abilities

Social Role
Projected attitudes and values

Self Image
Sense of self and worth

Traits
Why and how we behave in a certain way
Motives
What drives us, i.e. need for achievement, influence, affiliation

Figure 7.1 Personal Iceberg Metaphor Model Example.

Another interesting way to reflect on and consider your transferable skills comes from the work of Dick Bolles. His work on skills considers them under three categories: Personal, Transferable, and Work-related. He helps you to identify them by considering each category as your verbs, nouns, or adjectives:

Your particulate combination of skills is what makes you unique and can help you both sell yourself at interviews and support you in your own personal understanding and development.

Transferable Skills Brought to the Role by Potential Candidates

As we have referenced elsewhere, PPs come from a variety of backgrounds. Some may be coming straight from undergraduate degrees, others with years of experience in other roles, which may or may not be in health-related fields.

The list of potential transferable skills is long, and we would be unable to reference them all here; therefore, think of the list in Table 7.3 as a selection of examples:

Table 7.3 Skill types and examples

Skill Type		Description	Examples
Transferable functional skills	Verbs	These are your talents, gifts, and natural skills. There is often a preference to either people, data, or things	Driving, Communicating, Organising
Personal traits and skills	Adjectives	This can be seen to relate to your own self-discipline and management. It is the style in which you do your transferable skills	Dependable Accurate Punctual Kind Persistence
Work subject skills or knowledge skills	Nouns	These are your expertise, often learnt and developed over years	A subject, i.e., Psychology A second language IT, i.e., PowerPoint

Diverse Backgrounds

Coming from a non-Psychology graduate background, degree in English Literature and Women's Studies, working in physical rehab and end of life care before moving into mental health work, my aim at the beginning of my career was to a) get onto a PWP trainee course, and b) qualify! It wasn't until a few years later I started thinking about where I wanted my career to develop from there. I am now lucky enough to maintain a small clinical caseload alongside my role as a Team Lead in a Talking Therapies service, and my volunteer work in the British Association for Behavioural and Cognitive Psychotherapies (BABCP).

Sam Torney, National Health Service (NHS) Talking Therapies (TT) Team Lead, qualified Psychological Wellbeing Practitioner (PWP), and Chair of Low-Intensity Special Interest Group (LI-SIG), BABCP.

You do not have to have taken an undergraduate degree in psychology to train as a PP. Many non-psychological careers (e.g., teaching, nursing, social work, and retail) can equip individuals with and help them to develop and hone skills that are essential for those embarking on a career as a PP.

For example, a university undergraduate may bring familiarity with or have honed study skills, feel competent in researching for a topic or in their ability to reference in an essay.

A trainee PP who has previously trained and worked as a teacher will likely bring abilities in engaging people and conveying ideas. This may be beneficial and transferable in helping them to share interventions with clients or in being able to manage psycho educational groups.

An individual who has worked in a retail environment will have had the opportunity to develop skills in quickly building rapport and potentially in de-escalating conflict.

Many roles that have an element of working with people will support the development and value of 'soft skills' such as communication and empathy.

> Through a change of career direction from working as a builder to re-training and being employed part-time as a Person Centred Counsellor, I spotted the opportunity to apply for the role of trainee PWP. I thoroughly enjoyed my PWP training and went on to be employed as a PWP.
>
> Rob Leigh, NHS TT Supervision Lead, a qualified PWP, a High-intensity Cognitive Behavioural Therapist, and an Eye Movement Desensitisation and Reprocessing (EMDR) Consultant.

There are also many non-psychological roles that offer the opportunity to develop problem-solving skills, analytical thinking, and solution-focused approaches. What experiences and opportunities have you had that may demonstrate these types of skills?

> I am now in my early 40s and I came from a completely different profession, before deciding on a career in mental health. Thankfully, many of the skills developed in other jobs are transferrable to this role, including interpersonal communication, time management, computing, and administration skills.

I also have a diagnosis of ADHD which I worried could be a barrier to my career as a PP. However, I have found that thanks my ADHD I have been able to bring a creative side to the role, especially in adapting these interventions for individuals with vulnerabilities. Many of our service users have co-morbid learning difficulties, such as Autism and ADHD, and I find that, as a person who has his own life-long struggles, I am more relatable to them.

Adam Hope, Qualified Mental Health
Wellbeing Practitioner (MHWP)

It is acknowledged that having PPs in a team from a variety of backgrounds and experiences is valuable in both enhancing the skill sets in the team and in reflecting the communities they serve. This is further evidenced by the development of various routes into training (see Chapter 6).

Cultural Competence and Protected Characteristics

Cultural background and understanding are also key factors to consider here. What does your own cultural background mean to you, and what experiences has it given you?

Historically, psychological professions have not well represented the communities they serve. The psychological professions Workforce Census data shows that, in NHS TT for Anxiety and Depression (NHSTTad), we have made a little progress in this area with PP roles, but there is significant work still to do.

"Being Muslim from a South Asian background and having experienced mental health issues in my family, I wanted to ensure YP from different ethnic backgrounds, had someone they could relate too. There are not many people of colour within the mental health field, which is much needed as those from ethnic diverse communities, are at higher risk of developing mental health issues. There can be massive stigma within different cultures and communities and I wanted to make sure I could tap into this and create that awareness and understanding.

Minoritised communities can often be labelled as 'hard to reach' but in fact we, as mental health services, are hard for them to reach. I wanted to change this, bringing in my own experiences and culture, to help adapt my work with the YP. I would also ensure culture and race was discussed in all aspects of our work. I do sometimes feel that, if I don't say it, would another person who is White British mention this? This did and still does, sometimes feel a lot, as I cannot represent all my people and so, ensuring we are all comfortable in asking questions and being curious with working with YP from a different background to ourselves, is key. Some may feel awkward about it, which I understand but we need to start getting comfortable with being uncomfortable, this is how we grow. It has been going on for too long now and the system needs to change. I hope that I am part of that positive change.

Safa Asif, Qualified Children's Wellbeing
Practitioner (CWP)

In work commissioned by the Psychological Professions Network (PPN) to explore equality and diversity within the psychological professions, Margo Ononaiye led a project which has produced an Equality, Diversity, and Inclusion (EDI) resource bank and audit tool. These are hosted on the PPN website and provide an excellent starting point for exploring this wide-ranging topic. There are also some thought-provoking articles available on this subject, for example, Taf Kunorubwe and colleagues work on barriers to working in a culturally competent or culturally sensitive way in TT. Overall research in this area is providing evidence to show that improving our cultural awareness can aid better outcomes for clients.

Awareness of, and/or lived or living experience, with other protected characteristics, should also be considered here.

Social GGRRAAACCEEESSS is a framework, developed by John Burnham (2012), which allows us to consider our beliefs and prejudices in relation to our personal and social identity. It is important that we are aware of these in order to understand their impact on us both at an individual level, but also from a PP point of view, how they may show up in our practice, as issues relating to power and privilege.

Each of the individual aspects, as shown in Figure 7.2, may have its own impact, but it is also important to reflect on the issue

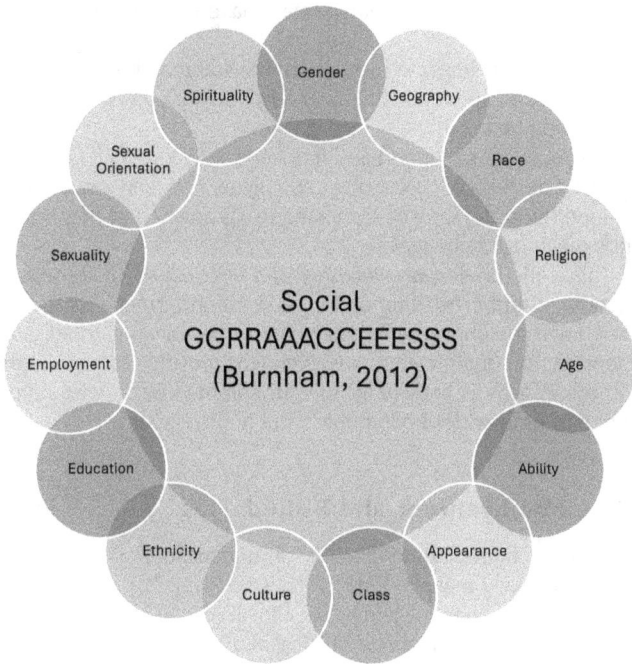

Figure 7.2   The Social GRRRAAACCEEESSS.

of intersectionality as well. This refers to where one individual may experience or be impacted by more than one aspect, creating their unique identity and experience.

Within EDI, there is also the concept of allyship. Being an ally is an active engagement of support and advocacy of positively utilising your own privilege to challenge discrimination, promote inclusion, and raise the voice of a marginalised group.

Cultural competence is about meeting the individual where they are rather than them having to meet us as services. It is about seeing the person, and if you have knowledge gaps, being curious.

Consider your awareness of your own position, whether that be your own experience of marginalisation or of privilege.

What do you bring with you?

What assumptions do others may make of you? And you of others?

How has this impacted you as an individual and how you act?

Does your experience help you advocate for others?

Can you be an ally?

Do you want to support and influence services?

If in a position of power due to privilege, how can you use this to understand the impact, for example, of policy and help influence meaningful change?

This is the briefest of overviews of a huge topic, so we would encourage further reading and consideration. Organisations are often keen to support recruitment from their locality, to support retention post qualification; however, what positive aspects might you bring, such as knowledge of your community, understanding of needs, or ideas for how to reach out and engage?

Time Management and Boundaries

In the busy, high-volume PP roles, an understanding of and ability to effectively manage time is also important. This could come through in diary management or the ability to effectively and appropriately contain a session or simply around being able to prioritise.

Having clear boundaries and being able to explain or implement these, be it service models and limitations of remit or other professional boundary considerations, is also a key skill.

These skills could be developed in many professional roles; however, as busy working mum's, the authors would also consider reflection on other areas or aspects of your life in which you may develop transferable skills, especially if personal circumstances, for example, caring responsibilities, managing childcare, or experience of mental health issues, have influenced your experiences.

Since my late Attention Deficit Hyperactivity Disorder (ADHD) diagnosis and autism diagnosis, I feel that my neurodivergence helps my practice. Now in my early 50s, the hypervigilance developed from years of being undiagnosed allows me to keenly observe body language, facial expressions, and intonation, helping me detect subtle cues from young people (YP) during sessions. This sensitivity aids in identifying discomfort or unease, prompting timely interventions.

My pattern recognition skills have been helpful in addressing avoidant behaviours and safeguarding concerns. As a trainee Educational Mental Health PP (EMHP), I increasingly find that I am seeing YP who are neurodivergent or suspected to be. My experiences enable me to recognize challenges, especially in females, that might be overlooked in busy school environments. Through supervision discussions, I've collaborated with schools to gain necessary support.

Louise Rawley, Qualified EMHP

Resilience and Adaptability

As we've mentioned, each individual will come with their own life experience; each journey is different and will come with its own challenges. How a person deals with these, and adapts or develops strategies to help them cope is important. This may be adaptability of thought or in behaviour. Being able to be flexible in how you approach or respond is an important skill.

As everyone is unique, how they relax or unwind and manage their own stress will be different. Whether it be physical exercise, family time, spirituality, or something different, knowing what you need for your own self care is an important skill in itself.

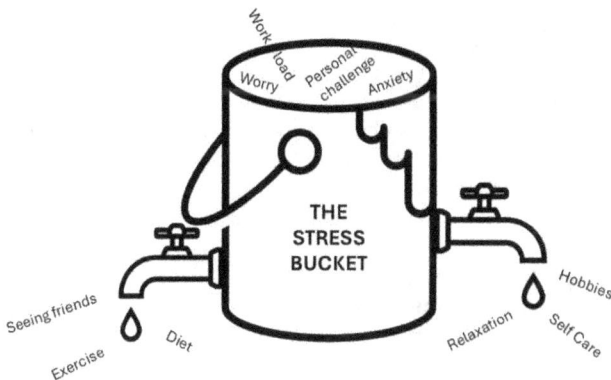

Figure 7.3 An Example of the Stress Bucket.

It might be useful to consider the 'Stress Bucket' as a way to understand and consider your own stress management capabilities and how you might apply these in a trainee or qualified PP role, with the competing personal, academic, and work-based demands.

Creativity

Although PPs work in very structured ways, often with manualised interventions, those with a creative background may feel surprised to hear that their creative skills can also be transferable and an advantage in the PP roles – for example, allowing them to build rapport, share ideas and materials, or communicate in accessible ways.

Interpersonal Communication

PPs are required to communicate with a range of different people. The first, most likely to come to mind is with your clients; however, you will also be required to communicate with peers, seniors, and those in management roles, both clinical and operational. There will also be a number of other stakeholders within and outside of your immediate team and/or organisation. Each different group will present with their own needs, as well as situations that you will need to adapt your communication skills and style for.

This will include your non-verbal and interpersonal skills. These may include, but are not limited to, active listening, rapport building, empathy, and non-verbal communication. In PWP literature, you may see the term 'common factor skills', which are further developed as part of their training and are therefore detailed further below.

The PP roles all focus on the individual, whether that is a CWP with a young person or a PWP with an older adult. All the PP roles will take a person-centred approach to an individual's care, collaborating with them to develop the treatment plan. There are many ways you could have developed these interpersonal and communication skills, in daily life with family, friends, and colleagues or maybe more formally, for example, a counselling skills course.

In addition to one-to-one interactions, you may find yourself needing to use these communicate skills in a group or meeting settings. There may also be situations, including in training where you need to present to an audience. Consider how you may need to adapt your style to meet the needs of these different situations?

While being empathetic and authentic is important, it is key that PPs are able to manage their own emotional responses and maintain professional boundaries. For example, clients may share things with their PP that may create an emotional response, but a PP will need to hold their own emotion in session and seek appropriate supervision or peer support after.

The Art of Feedback

Giving and being able to receive (and act) on feedback is an important skill. This may be within teaching, supervision, or personal reflection. In all cases, it is important that feedback is constructive, in order to support growth and development. This could apply to both personal and professional development.

PPs may have developed skills in giving and receiving feedback, for example, if they have had roles supporting or managing staff in a previous role.

Technology

Technology of many descriptions is a very fast-paced development in health care at present. There had been a gradual shift to increasing use of technology, for example, electronic records, PWP training in completing assessments via the telephone, not all contacts face to face, and early versions of computerised cognitive behavioural therapy (cCBT); however, the COVID pandemic accelerated the move towards increasing use of technology.

Now, as well as the transferable skills and competence in basic IT literacy skills, such as Word, confidence in other forms of technology is also an asset to the PP. Below are some examples of how technology is increasingly being incorporated into health care; therefore, consider how your current levels of IT skills and experience could be useful in a PP role.

The use of software such as MS Teams and NHS Attend Anywhere to provide audio and visual connection with clients for 1:1 appointments or group delivery was a significant shift in the pandemic and is now commonplace, offering clients increasing choice in how they access their health care provision. Platforms, such as Teams, have also supported the development of contact between teams and wider system colleagues, increasing options and flexibility for meetings and networking. Do you have experience of effectively using this kind of software?

The market of digital interventions, such as cCBT and online resources, has also increased considerably with a range of private provider companies and individuals, as well as some NHS-commissioned services developing their own in-house support packages and materials.

The most recent developments focus on artificial intelligence (AI)-driven technology. In the mental health field, these are things such as 'digital front doors' with AI-assisted triages, programmes that are using chatbots to support triage questioning and data set completion, with some also developing resources to also support clients whilst waiting or between sessions in treatment.

Charlotte Temple, a specialist lecturer on CWP and EMHP programmes, also highlighted to us another area of development, Spectrum Gaming, a Manchester-based service, providing online community provision for autistic young people. Other MHWPs also referenced the use of new technology, including trials involving Virtual Reality. These are just two examples; it is a fast-paced area of development and research.

Consider your own confidence in accessing and utilising online programmes and materials; are you able to check and understand if something is from a credible source, and are you able to support and explain programmes and apps to others (this could be currently in non-mental health contexts)?

One thing we do know is with current policy and commercial drivers, this field is going to continue to grow and develop; therefore, if you are able to bring some IT literacy with you or have the skills in adapting to new tech tools and innovations, this will be very beneficial.

In addition, there is the consideration of the data, often collected within IT systems. This can include data such as clinical measures and attendance. Being able to understand, interpret, and utilise this data in services with key performance indicators may also be important in roles, particularly as careers progress.

Collaboration and Building Networks

Although as PPs you are registered as individuals, these roles cannot be delivered effectively in silo. As stipulated in the registration guidance, PPs must work in a system of care.

There will be team working with your immediate colleagues, for example, PWPs working together to deliver a psychoeducational group or with a high-intensity therapy colleague to step a client up within the team.

There will also be occasions where you may work with other professional colleagues in a Multidisciplinary Team (MDT) to discuss and plan care for a client, for example, in the role of an MHWP in a Community Mental Health Team or a Children's Wellbeing Practitioner in a Child and Adolescent Mental Health Team, where the MDT approach is key to ensuring holistic practice and the best outcomes for the client.

There are also examples of collaboration with other systems of care, social care, education system, and other health care teams, for example, the work of EMHPs in the delivery of the Whole School Approach programme or PWPs in long-term conditions pathways, co-locating with physical health colleagues.

As careers develop (Chapters 12 and 13), there may be an opportunity or a need to network wider, to share good practice, build partnerships, contribute or provide feedback to more senior colleagues about policy, or to promote services to the wider public. This list is not exhaustive, and it is worth reflecting on skills, attributes and experiences that you may have to support you in this networking and collaborative approach.

Transferable Skills Developed through the Training and Role Itself

Within all of the PP training courses, there are skills which are both taught academically and then also learnt and honed on the job. Many of these skill groups are detailed above, as they could also be brought by the PP from previous experiences; however, it is important to ensure that they are being applied appropriately within the context of the PP role and that you continue to develop and consolidate skills and competencies throughout your training and qualified life.

Common Factor Skills

In PWP literature, you may see the term 'common factor skills'; this term is not used explicitly in Children and Young People's courses, but these interpersonal skills can be seen as broadly transferable between all of the PP roles. Although many of those applying for PP courses will identify with many of these characteristics pre-application, they are further developed in the training year.

They include having a positive, non-judgemental attitude, as clients are all individuals and will come with many different experiences and beliefs. There are also a range of non-verbal competences, so PPs should consider and appropriately use eye contact, facial expression, and posture. Consideration should also be given to environmental factors such as seating arrangements.

In addition, there are the verbal competences, as PP interventions are often referred to under the banner of 'talking therapies' (NHSTTad) or manualised approaches (CYP), people can get caught up in the verbal aspects, which is why in training there is a specific focus on non-verbal interpersonal skills. However, competent use of our verbal skills is required to ensure that we communicate with clients effectively and collaboratively for positive outcomes. These include paraphrasing, reflection, empathy, summarising, and providing factually accurate and realistic reassurance.

Ethical Practice

In Chapter 9, professional ethics are discussed in detail; however, this is also relevant to transferable skills, so important to reference here. Courses will teach PPs the core competencies of their role and remit and how to apply these.

Practicing ethically requires us to develop and integrate values into our practice. Many NHS or provider organisations will also align their mission and objectives to values. These include integrity, accountability, respect and dignity, compassion, and a commitment to improving lives through quality care. We need to reflect on how we incorporate these values into our thought processes, behaviours, and decision-making in practice.

On qualification, PPs are required to complete registration for their profession, which commits them to upholding the values and competencies of their specific role.

As well as practicing ethically, within their competencies and values, PP roles also require us to be professionals within our organisations. Professionalism considers our appearance, approach, and how we conduct our practice. As such, thought and care should be placed in how we show up as ourselves in our roles.

In turn, we can and should apply many of these principles in our everyday lives, and as such, they are transferable skills.

Active Listening

Listening is a skill, not just hearing the words but understanding them in their context and meaningful responding. It helps us to develop a rapport and improved communication, ensuring that we understand the speaker, their meaning, intent, and perspective.

Risk Assessment

This is a core skill within the PP roles and training. Each PP training provider will teach and assess this skill on the course. Employing services will then have policy, procedures, and ongoing training in place to ensure clinical competency.

In April 2025, NHS England published staying safe from suicide guidance, which provides detailed best practice in regards to assessment, formulation, and management of risk. The guidance was designed to be holistic and person-centred and marks a move away from risk prediction toward managing safety.

Diary Management

We have already referenced above time management. Diary management requires this but also incorporates additional skills. As a trainee, you will be introduced to your employer's system for clinical record keeping, and many of these systems also function as appointment booking and PP diaries. Commonly used systems include IAPTUS, PCMIS, and RIO.

You will be supported through line management and case management supervision with your job plan; however, the day-to-day management of this will be your responsibility, ensuring that you meet your clinical hours by ensuring you have enough client assessments and treatments booked in, writing up your clinical notes in the required timeframes, and considering the timings of other requirements such as supervision and meetings. There may also be other ad hoc requirements that require you to adjust your diary, for example, services running events for Mental Health Awareness Week.

In high-volume work, being organised is key; some PPs find it helpful to set reminders or have templates for certain tasks. Always remember to ask line managers or supervisors for tips and support early; don't let yourself become overwhelmed.

Clinical Record Keeping

As registered PPs, our employers and governing bodies require us to keep accurate clinical records for our clients.

Clinical note writing is a skill that requires practice. Notes need to be concise, accurate, and written in a timely manner.

All organisations will have expected standards and guidance; some will also provide specific templates.

PPs should also be aware of the BABCP Standards of Conduct, Performance, and Ethics and the British Psychological Society Fitness to Practice Framework in relation to record keeping.

From PP to Educator

In Chapter 13, we discuss transitioning from clinical PP roles to roles in academia, that is, lecturer, in more detail; however, it is also a transferable skill that could be seen to be gained through training and clinical practice, so it is covered here briefly too.

In training, you are taught to deliver guided self-help or manualised interventions to clients. These skills in delivering interventions are further enhanced as you develop in practice. These skills could be seen as educational in supporting clients to become their own therapist, by learning tools and interventions to manage their symptoms.

The transferable educator and presentation skills are also gained and developed through delivering CPD to colleagues or training or information to colleagues, from non-psychological backgrounds.

Leadership in Psychological Practice

Throughout this book, there are references to teamwork, collaboration, and supervision. Managing group dynamics, conflict resolution, peer support, and navigating teams can all aid the development of leadership skills over time.

Elspeth and Kirsty like the idea of leadership at all levels; the NHS is biodimensional in its leadership structure, requiring achievement of targets, as well as vision for change. PPs have value, skill, and a voice that, when appropriate, can support these aims.

These leadership skills can be used in role or as transitioning from a PP role to other leadership and management roles in health care (or other industries).

Reflection

A key skill as a PP is the ability to reflect. This process of self-observation and self-evaluation is done independently or within a supervisory environment. Clinically, it is a process that requires us to think deeply about past experience (Bennett-Levy, Thwaites, Chaddock, & Davis, 2009) and consider the implications of decisions made and actions taken, in more detail (Moon, 1999).

Reflexivity takes this continual reflective process and incorporates self-awareness. It allows you to then analytically assess your practice and to develop insights, helping you to develop and improve yourself and your practice. It is an active and individual process that should culminate in a personal development plan or actions.

There are multiple models and frameworks that can be used to support you in your reflective practice, for example, Gibbs (1988) or Rolfe, Freshwater, and Jasper (2001).

You will need to be able to use this skill, to apply for training, during training, as a qualified PP in both sessions and supervision and in your development. Reflecting on your own skills is a chance to practice your ability to reflect on yourself, your situation, values, and behaviours.

In addition, as you progress in your career, you can utilise reflection to support your decision-making processes for next steps, transitions, or lateral moves. Incorporating ideas such as 'The Growth Mindset', more information on Scope for Growth can also be found on the South West NHS Leadership Academy website. These personal reflections can then also be linked into Line Management conversation and to guide CPD choices and opportunities.

Having now read through this chapter, take a moment to reconsider the question posed at the beginning – what skills do you already possess which will aid you as a PP? How have you developed these?

Table 7.4 Having read Chapter 7, this is an opportunity to reflect again on your transferable skills

Transferable Skill	Evidenced by

Box 7.1 References and wider reading

Bennett-Levy, J., Thwaites, R., Chaddock, C., & Davis, M. (2009). The role of cognitive-behavioural therapy in the treatment of anxiety disorders. *Journal of Anxiety Disorders*, 23 (5), pp. 675–684.

Bolles, R.N. (2019). *What colour is your parachute? A practical manual for job-hunters and career-changers.* Ten Speed Press.

British Association of Cognitive and Behavioural Psychotherapies. (2022). *Standards of conduct, performance, and ethics.* BABCP.

British Psychological Society. (2022). *Wider psychological workforce (WPW) register: Fitness to practice framework.* BPS.

Burnham, J. (2012). Developments in social GRRRAAAC-CEEESSS: Visible-invisible and voiced-unvoiced. In I.-B. Krause (Ed.), *Culture and reflexivity in systemic psychotherapy: Mutual perspectives* (pp. 139–160). Karnac Books.

Gibbs, G. (1988). *Learning by doing: A guide to teaching and learning methods.* Further Education Unit, Oxford Polytechnic.

Kunorubwe, T., Edwards, A., & Santhosh, S. (2022). The struggles of working in a culturally competent or culturally sensitive way within IAPT: Part 1. *CBT Today.* September 2022.

Moon, R. (1999). *The art of learning.* Learning Press.

NHS England. (2025). *Psychological professions national workforce census.* NHS England. https://www.england. nhs.uk/publication/psychological-professions-workforce-census/

NHS England. (2025). *Staying safe from suicide.* NHS England.

Rolfe, G., Freshwater, D., & Jasper, M. (2001). *Critical reflection in nursing and the helping professions.* Palgrave Macmillan.

Chapter 8

Being a Trainee

There are a range of routes that can be taken to train as a psychological practitioner (PP). This chapter gives an overview of the routes, some of the main elements of training, and includes the voices of PPs across the roles sharing their experiences of this intense but rewarding year.

Training

Training to be a PP typically takes 12 months to complete as a full-time programme. Full time is the most common method of completing this training, although there are some part-time options available. The academic element of training is supported by a clinical practice placement and regular clinical supervision.

Notably, 12 months is not a long duration, and it would be remiss not to note that, as well as being highly rewarding, the training year is intense.

Kelly DeSantis, a qualified Psychological Wellbeing Practitioner (PWP), tells us that their training year was "interesting, rewarding, but also exhausting, especially when you are working full time and have a family". They do go on to say that the year overall was 'very positive', adding, "I am glad I did it and I enjoyed it overall, but I did have to learn the importance of balance and boundaries!".

Anne Masterson, a qualified Children's Wellbeing Practitioner (CWP), describes their training year as 'intensive but enjoyable' and says that they are glad they completed the training because they love their job. As a recently qualified practitioner, they also note that they are excited by the future and what is to come.

DOI: 10.4324/9781003542049-8

Louise Rawley, a qualified Education Mental Health Practitioner (EMHP), describes the year as 'very full-on', with lots to try and take in. They note that the course itself is challenging. However, they also say that they are grateful to have had the opportunity to train as they have never had a job that gives them 'as much purpose as this one does'.

Kirsten Brown, a qualified Mental Health Wellbeing Practitioner (MHWP), tells us, "I was in heaven on my training year, as the course encompassed everything I have wanted to study for years". They acknowledge how challenging the year was but say that "the help and support I had around me was so valuable, as at times I needed to lean on others. The training is set up so that you can and should do this". They are keen to point out what a rewarding role theirs is.

There are distinct courses for each of the PP roles, and it is important to note that these are not interchangeable. If you complete training as a PWP, for example, you will be eligible to register and work as a PWP with an adult population and within a specified system of care. The PWP qualification would not train you in the required competencies to be able to work and register as an MHWP, a CWP, or an EMHP working with children and young people (YP).

Across the four main PP roles, there are options to complete the qualification at an undergraduate or postgraduate level. For the PWP role, which has been around the longest, there are now

Table 8.1 Training routes for PPs

Role	Training Routes
PWP	PWP-specific university training course as undergraduate (level 6) or postgraduate (level 7)
	PWP university training as part of a wider programme of study as undergraduate (level 6) or postgraduate (level 7)
	Apprenticeship (level 6)
MHWP	MHWP-specific university training course as undergraduate (level 6) or postgraduate (level 7)
CWP	CWP-specific university training course as undergraduate (level 6) or postgraduate (level 7)
EMHP	EMHP-specific university training course as undergraduate (level 6) or postgraduate (level 7)

also apprenticeship routes available – we'll talk about these a little more further into this chapter.

The broad training route options available are detailed in Table 8.1.

Funding

Training in any of the PP roles is usually funded by the National Health Service (NHS). This means that, in most cases, it is the NHS that covers the cost of the training course, as well as your salary during the training year, and not the organisation where you are placed.

Since 1 April 2022, there has been a two-year psychological professions funding rules policy implemented. This means that anyone who starts an NHS-funded psychological therapies training course must wait two years following the expected completion date of that training (whether they fully complete it or not) before they can begin a further NHS-funded training course.

The overall aim of the funding rule is to ensure that public money is well spent, and that trained practitioners are then able to use those skills they have been trained in and deliver services that are required to meet the growing need and demand for psychological treatment. The requirement of staying in a particular role for a period following training also has the benefit of ensuring new skills and ways of working can be embedded, benefiting you as a PP as well.

PWP Apprenticeships

A report from Health Education England (HEE, now merged with NHS England) in 2019 made recommendations that alternative types of PWP training should be implemented, including "more flexible courses that could train people who would benefit from longer training and apprenticeship and vocational training routes".

One of the aims of this was to increase access into the role for people in the local communities and from diverse demographic backgrounds. We know, from research, that historically psychological professions have not well represented the communities they serve. In the report to HEE, it was noted that "The hope was that a supported route into training through apprenticeship processes could facilitate a home-grown workforce to emerge that could potentially produce a more representative and stable workforce in the future".

The PWP apprenticeship route was approved for delivery in 2019 and continues to run successfully. It is not necessarily that different to the under- and postgraduate routes in content or requirements, simply a different pathway. PWPs who have qualified via the apprenticeship route can work and register the same as PWPs trained otherwise.

As a PWP apprentice, you work towards achieving a specified range of knowledge, skills, and behaviours (KSBs), as set out in the occupational standards. You will develop these KSBs through practice in the work placement and additional training (education). When you are consistently demonstrating the ability to work at or above the level set out in the occupational standards, this is deemed as meeting occupational competency.

A requirement of apprenticeship positions is that an English and mathematics qualification to level 2 must be achieved. If you do not have this at the beginning of training, you must undertake this "functional skills qualification" alongside the PWP work. You must achieve the English and mathematics qualifications, as what is called a gateway requirement, before being able to undertake the end-point assessment and complete the PWP qualification. (It is called a gateway requirement, as you must have it before you can move on through the 'gate'!)

There are not yet apprenticeship routes into the other PP roles of CWP, EMHP, or MHWP.

Curricula

A curriculum refers to the overall programme and processes for delivering it, and there is a distinct curriculum for each of the PP training programmes. There are numerous assessment requirements or competencies to demonstrate in order to achieve the relevant qualification as a PP, regardless of the type of qualification, and the national curricula lay these out in detail.

National curricula may be implemented in slightly differing ways by different higher education institutions (HEIs), for example, in the way that modules and credits are broken down (i.e., some education providers may split the content over more or fewer modules than listed in the curriculum), or in the way in which assignments are structured or linked to learning outcomes. However, the broad areas and requirements for training courses are set out by the national curricula. The modules are summarised in Table 8.2.

Table 8.2 PP training course module breakdowns

PP Role	National Curriculum Modules
Psychological Wellbeing Practitioner	Module 1 – Engagement and assessment of patients with common mental health problems
	Module 2 – Evidence-based low-intensity treatment for common mental health disorders
	Module 3 – Values, diversity, and context
Mental Health Wellbeing Practitioner	Module 1 – Engagement and assessment with people with severe mental health problems
	Module 2 – Care planning in partnership
	Module 3 – Wellbeing-focused psychologically-informed interventions for severe mental health problems
Children's Wellbeing Practitioner	Module 1 – Children and YP's mental health settings: Context and values
	Module 2 – Assessment and engagement
	Module 3 – Evidence-based interventions for common mental health problems with children and YP: Theory and skills
	Module 4 – Working, assessing, and engaging in community-based and primary care settings
	Module 5 – Mental health prevention in community and primary care settings
	Module 6 – Interventions for emerging mental health difficulties in community and primary care settings
Education Mental Health Practitioner	Module 1 – Children and YP's mental health settings: context and values
	Module 2 – Assessment and engagement
	Module 3 – Evidence-based interventions for common mental health problems with children and YP: Theory and skills
	Module 4 – Working, assessing, and engaging in education settings
	Module 5 – Common problems and processes in education settings
	Module 6 – Interventions for emerging mental health difficulties in education settings

Within each module, the curriculum will set out a range of learning objectives (LOs). These break down what knowledge, understanding, and skills you should have achieved on completion of the module. The teaching content for that module will be aligned to the LOs, and any submissions of work for that module should give the opportunity for the LOs to be assessed.

Service Placements and Clinical Practice

One of the things (certainly in our opinion, as authors and practitioners) that stands out about PP training is the combination of theoretical learning alongside the opportunity to do the job in your clinical practice placement. We're not alone in our thinking here either.

Amy Newton, a qualified CWP, tells us, "The best thing about the training course was the ability to put theory into practice straight away. The course and the clinical practice went hand in hand".

Lettie Smyth, a qualified CWP and supervisor, shares that

Although I had worked with children and young adults previously, I learned so much during my training about how to practice clinically, reflecting on the nuances of this. Although the year was intense, the aspect of it being run as a recruit to train programme really allowed my learning to feel tangible. I could see it play out in practice as a process of development and progress.

A key part of training courses across the PP roles is placement within a clinical service and the opportunity to hold a caseload. In most cases, the service will be your direct employer throughout the training year, with attendance at teaching and study days, and completion of the course, incorporated into your working hours and a condition of your contract.

The hope would then be for you to continue with the service as a qualified PP once your training year is over, although it should be noted that funding for this is not always guaranteed, and the ability to implement this may vary across services.

As a trainee PP, you will be working within a service that is relevant to the role in which you are being trained. For example:

- PWPs will be placed in NHS Talking Therapies for Anxiety and Depression services.
- MHWPs will be placed in Community Mental Health Teams or other services supporting adults with severe mental health difficulties.
- CWPs will be placed in Children and Young People's Mental Health Services, with links and connections to community-based organisations and venues.
- EMHPs will be placed in Mental Health Support Teams with connections to schools, colleges, and education providers.

During your training year, your job role and main purpose will be training as a PP, and therefore, your job plan and main duties should reflect this and align with the course requirements. You should be supernumerary, meaning that you are an additional member of staff to the team, rather than completing an additional job role alongside your training. Your training *is* your job role for the year and believe us when we say (from experience!) that there is plenty to do for this to fill your working hours.

It may be that your service has opportunities for you to get involved in observing or supporting any wider offer or the practice of other practitioners, particularly in the early period before you have begun picking up a caseload of your own. However, this would be with the purpose of embedding you in the service and helping you understand the offer, giving you additional learning opportunities via observation, rather than being a core part of your job role.

For example, as a CWP, you may have the opportunity to join a community-based fun day or summer holiday provision for children and YP in the local area, as an extra pair of hands and to observe how other staff from your placement service operate and engage with the community. As a PWP, you may have the opportunity to join an assessment or treatment session in another modality of therapy offered within the service, such as high-intensity cognitive behavioural therapy (CBT), as an observer. It can be incredibly beneficial to take up these opportunities, to get a wider experience of the mental health offer in your local area, and to see other practitioners in action. You can pick up a broader understanding of support options or ways of working that will enhance your own practice as you begin with your own caseload.

Supervision

Clinical supervision, offered regularly and at a high frequency, is an important part of the training year to become a PP.

Faye Whitehill, a qualified CWP, tells us that it was great to have someone with experience and knowledge of the role giving them one-to-one support and a safe space to discuss cases and any personal anxieties they had about what they were delivering. Their supervisor helped them set actions and plan to move forward and develop. Faye also notes that having a consistent person for this across the year helped build their confidence in supervision. Faye tells us, "Knowing that any issues that come up, or struggles you are having will be heard and normalised helps you relax into the training year".

Melissa Street is a Consultant Psychological Therapist for a Child and Adolescent Mental Health Service (CAMHS), an employer of CWPs, and a former Programme Lead for a CWP training programme. She notes the benefits of having supervisor support during training, particularly in keeping up to date with paperwork and course requirements. She says, "Working alongside your supervisor to keep up to date with the requirements of the course is best, and this helps ensure you don't end up behind".

Clinical supervision is separate and in addition to line management supervision (LMS) that will, in most cases, be provided to all employees. Where LMS can generally be provided by anyone in a management position, clinical supervision must be provided by an appropriately qualified, experienced practitioner who usually also has training in CBT-informed practice.

Clinical supervision takes two forms:

- Clinical Case Management Supervision
  This is focused on reviewing the caseload of the trainee PP. There is a clear structure around order cases that are presented and the level of detail covered. This allows the supervisor to ensure that the trainee is holding a suitably sized caseload,

with the appropriate types of cases, and that the interventions being offered are in line with the remit of the role and the training received.

- Clinical Skills Supervision* (CSS)
  This is focused on developing the skills of the trainee PP. This can be done through methods such as watching recordings of clinical practice for the purpose of reflection, practicing skills through role-play or other activities, and discussion. CSS is generally provided in group format, allowing trainees to learn from one another and engage in skills practice activities with peers as well as the supervisor.

*It should be noted that, for MHWPs, CSS is often referred to as psychological intervention supervision (PIS), including in the NHS role-specific guidance document "Mental Health Wellbeing Practitioner: A Guide to Practice". The format of PIS is broadly similar to CSS; however, some specific elements of MHWP supervision are covered in more detail in the role-specific chapter of this book (see Chapter 3 – Being a Mental Health Wellbeing Practitioner).

During the training year, the frequency of clinical supervision is specified within course curricula. The frequency is high to support development across the intense 12 months of training, supplementing the learning that takes place in teaching and ensuring that trainees are practicing safely and competently. The amount of supervision that is required for a trainee PP is detailed in Table 8.3.

Qualified EMHP Louise Rawley identifies one of the benefits of supervision as being that it allowed them to better grasp things they'd not fully understood during teaching.

Table 8.3 Supervision requirements for trainee PPs

Type of Supervision	Format	Frequency	Duration
Clinical case management	Individual	Weekly	60 minutes minimum
Clinical skills	Group Max. four people for PWP/CWP/EMHP Max. three people for MHWP	Fortnightly	30 minutes per person minimum

Lauren White, a qualified CWP, says that when they originally started supervision, they questioned everything they were doing and if it was right. However, with the support of their supervisor, by the end of the year, they had developed confidence in their choices and the interventions they were delivering.

The experiences noted above are common themes identified by trainee PPs and highlight the benefits and importance of supervision within the training year, in particular. Due to trainees who access these courses often coming to them with some level of previous experience working in a mental health, psychology, education, or other people focused settings, when they begin to learn a new way of working with people for their PP role, it can lead to feeling suddenly aware of how much they don't know or need to learn across the year.

Adam Hope, a qualified MHWP, tells us that their previous experience of supervision was that it was limited in frequency and delivered over the phone. They tell us that supervision in their MHWP role has been "much more frequent, focused, and structured". Adam tells us,

> Supervision within this role is highly valued and is considered an important part of professional development. At times the role can be emotionally demanding, and supervision provides the opportunity to reflect on your own wellbeing and be supported with this.

Melissa Street (who we met earlier) spoke to us about the benefit of building a good supervisory relationship and being open and transparent in supervision. She says,

> You don't have to only show your best side to your supervisor, it's important to be honest about areas you're struggling with as well as sharing the areas you're doing well in. Although this might feel tricky it certainly gives your supervisor the best opportunity to support you in developing your understanding, skills, and practice.

Reflection and Reflective Practice

A key thread that is woven through PP training courses is that of reflection, supporting all PPs to become effective reflective practitioners. Reflective practice is broadly understood, across a wide range of roles, to refer to the ability to look back on an experience and pick out key learning from this, supported by critical evaluation of theory and literature that can help make sense of the experience, with the aim of identifying actions that can be carried forward to enhance and improve practice in the future.

This is the same with PP roles and training, where practitioners are encouraged to actively think about what happened (in the assessment, treatment session, groupwork, or wider aspect of work), why that might have happened, what was good or not so good about it, and how this can inform what is done in the future.

Melissa Street (who we met earlier) notes that "Reflection is a skill. To some people this comes more naturally but it's a skill that you need to work on".

The skill of reflecting is something that can be worked on individually, will be encouraged via assignments during training, and can be integrated into clinical supervision with the support of your supervisor and peers.

Teaching

Teaching during PP courses is usually scheduled over one or two days per week. There may be some variation in this across different HEIs. For example, some courses will consistently have two days of teaching every week across the training year, whereas others may 'front load' some of the teaching with blocks of three, four, or five days in teaching per week at the very start of the course, and others may vary across the terms. Teaching will generally cover three terms, with breaks in between and sometimes 'reading weeks' added in for self-directed study.

Different PP roles and different HEIs may have different starting times for courses across the year, with September or January being common points for intake.

Teaching on PP courses will take the form of theoretical learning, through lectures or workshops, for example, and specific skills practice sessions with the education provider. This is often supported further by practice-based learning, which is the completion of directed learning activities within the service placement part of the role. These practice-based learning activities may include shadowing or observation of clinical practice, role-play or group practice activities with peers, individual practice activities and reflection, or problem-based learning activities.

Lecturers and tutors who deliver teaching for PP training are required, by the body that accredits courses, the British Psychological Society, to have the necessary knowledge, experience, and skill to support trainees' learning and development of clinical competence. Those who demonstrate this mix most often come from roles within clinical psychology, high-intensity CBT practice, or are low-intensity CBT-informed PPs (i.e., PWPs, CWPs, or EMHPs) themselves.

Due to how new the MHWP course is, there may not yet be MHWPs with sufficient clinical experience to move into MHWP educator roles. However, this likely will come with time, following the precedent of the other PP courses.

Types of Assignments

Across the graduate and postgraduate training courses, there will be several formal assessments completed that will need to be passed for overall completion and qualification as a PP. Assignments will be linked to specific course modules and LOs, drawn from the national curriculum guidance for courses, as outlined above.

Due to variances across different training providers (HEIs), it is not possible to give specific details here; however, we can give an overview of the types of assignments that are likely to be included.

- Recordings of clinical practice
  Due to the practical nature of PP courses, where you are learning the role alongside theory, most courses require submissions of recordings of clinical practice. This will involve recording a full assessment or treatment session that has been completed with a client and submitting this to be reviewed and marked against specific criteria. Most commonly, this would be a video recording; however, there may be some courses or occasions where audio-only recordings are utilised.

  It is, of course, imperative that appropriate informed consent has been gained from any client who is appearing in the recording. Individual courses and services will have consent forms and processes for managing this.

- Reflective write-ups
  To accompany recordings of clinical practice, it is common for you to be asked to write a reflective piece. This gives the opportunity to identify areas of strength and areas for further development within the recorded session. For example, you might identify that you did a good job setting an agenda, but your use of summarising could benefit from further development. You can then identify what you have learnt from the experience, link this to theory and literature, and set actions to develop your practice going forward. This type of assignment will usually be submitted at the same time as the clinical recording.
- Observed Structured Clinical Examination (OSCE)
  An OSCE is a clinical simulation used to assess your clinical skills performance and competencies in a scenario situation. It can commonly be used to assess the ability to conduct assessments, deliver low-intensity interventions, or manage care. Where assessment strategies based on real clinical practice (such as submission of clinical practice recordings) can produce variance in experience across the trainees in a cohort, the benefit of an OSCE is the standardised experience, meaning that all trainees are assessed in the same way.
- Case reports
  A case report is a written assignment that gives you the opportunity to demonstrate in-depth understanding of a case from your clinical practice. The case will be presented anonymously (using no names, or clearly stating a pseudonym from the start) and give detailed information about elements such as the assessment, the identified presenting problem, the formulation, the rationale for chosen intervention, the intervention and content of clinical work, the overall outcome for the case and routine outcome measure scoring, and often your closing reflections on the experience of the case overall. Case reports will generally require reference to underpinning theory and literature to be included throughout, to demonstrate your ability to make theory-to-practice links.
- Essays
  Essays may be used as assessment strategies to test your knowledge of specific elements linked to the role and psychological practice, or to demonstrate the ability to critically appraise literature and theoretical content. These will be more linked to

theoretical learning and associated LOs than, for example, a case report.

- Reports
  You may be required to complete reports, which are stylistically different from essay submissions, to demonstrate your effectiveness in delivering wider aspects of the role. For example, EMHPs may be required to write reports detailing school audits, delivery of psychoeducation, or groupwork delivery; CWPs may be required to write reports detailing their delivery of staff training.

- Presentations
  Presentations, delivered either individually or as part of a group assignment, may be used as assessment strategies. Delivering presentations will not only demonstrate theoretical learning and ability to make theory-to-practice links but also develop wider, transferable skills relevant to the role. This might include the ability to speak to a group, the ability to succinctly deliver information in a timed situation, or the ability to develop slides and resources to support understanding.

- Examinations
  Written formal examinations may be used to test you on knowledge of the role and module content. The format of exams can vary across training providers, for example, using brief answer questions or longer form, essay-style answers.

- Portfolio Document
  PP training courses, due to their nature of combining theoretical learning and clinical practice, often require submission of a portfolio completed across the training year that demonstrates development of the required skills and competencies. The portfolio document, in some instances, is a requirement for completion of the course (meaning that it must be present and signed off as complete) but not a formal submission (which might receive a mark or grade).

- Practice Skills Assessment Document (PSAD)
  A PSAD is similar in nature to a portfolio, in that it is a document that evidences required competencies developed in clinical practice.

Matthew Draper is a current trainee on a CWP course and spoke to us about the assignments, saying, "There are some challenging aspects to the assignments, but nothing beyond what you would expect from a postgraduate diploma".

Ally Boyne is a specialist lecturer and marking coordinator on EMHP and CWP programmes, and a CBT therapist. She tells us,

> All of the assignments you will engage with across the programme will be designed to support PPs and their practice. All the training providers work hard to liaise with stakeholders and service leads to ensure the assignments are designed with the role in mind and remain relevant to the role and the changing landscape of the settings you will be delivering across.

Trainee Experience

As your authors, we wanted to ensure that we gave opportunity in this chapter for you to hear from trainees who have completed, or are currently completing, PP training courses. The experiences below hopefully acknowledge some of the challenges of training, whilst also demonstrating how beneficial the year can be.

Ellie McKelvey, a current trainee CWP, speaks highly of her experience so far, saying

> My favourite part of the training is the teaching. The lecturers are so helpful. I didn't particularly enjoy my undergraduate experience and never felt comfortable speaking out in lectures or tutorials. Because of my cohort and lecturers now, I feel comfortable and confident discussing my thoughts, experiences, and opinions on the content we're learning. The group are friendly and supportive especially during presentations and assessments. The peer feedback and words of encouragement are invaluable.

Louise Rawley is a qualified EMHP. As someone who is neurodivergent, having had a late diagnosis in adulthood, she identifies that, during the training year, the number of new experiences, different settings, different people, and changes to manage in a relatively short space of time was uniquely challenging. Louise believes, having now completed the training, that her neurodivergence makes her a better practitioner given that lived and living experience.

However, Louise also says, quite honestly, that the course was "one of the hardest things I've ever done". She is quick to add that the course tutors were supportive, that she was lucky to work as part of a 'fantastic' MHST, and that she had encouraging supervisors who made difficult times a lot easier.

Sophie Maylor, a qualified CWP, spoke to us about how she came to the training course as a non-graduate. Sophie had lots of experience working with children, YP, and families, and had previously been a clinical support worker in a CAMHS team. The CWP course felt like 'the perfect fit' for Sophie and was where she wanted to develop her career, and she was ecstatic to secure a place based on her experience and enthusiasm for the role, without having an undergraduate degree.

Sophie describes herself as someone who will 'throw myself into anything' but did, quite frankly, share that she had some trepidation in joining a cohort of trainees who, in some cases, had much more academic experience. Sophie admits that the academic side of the programme was the more challenging aspect for her. She shares, "I realised that I was quite confident and comfortable in the clinical work, working with young people and parents, but I needed to build my academic skills. That was the part that was more difficult for me".

Sophie shares that reaching out for support, from her service manager, clinical supervisor, and course tutor, was helpful. They supported her to take the knowledge 'out of my head and put it onto paper'. She also feels that she really benefited from having the practical work, the CWP practice, alongside the learning and theory. "The practical work kept me going", Sophie tells us, sharing that this was backed up by a high score she achieved on a clinical recording submission, motivating her to carry on.

Sandi McGuire, a qualified CWP, came to the training having had an established career already, with around 20 years in her previous job in the prison service. Sandi had left that role wanting a career change and decided that working with children was where she wanted to be. She self-funded some further training but found that this didn't directly help her get into a job role. Sandi says, of the CWP course, "It's a great way in".

Paula Mohin is a trainee CWP and shares her experience. She says, "I find the interactions with other trainees interesting as we all have different experiences that can add things to our bank of knowledge, and it supports a positive environment".

Matthew Draper (who we met earlier) backs this up, saying "I enjoy learning from my peers on the course, who all come from a range of backgrounds with a wealth of experience that, when shared, offers us all the chance to grow and develop".

Matthew also adds,

> The tutors on my course are passionate about the topics they deliver and make me feel very supported. Feedback is actioned and discussed from session to session, making the course seem like a shared journey that the tutors help me on and not just a solo journey where they are signposting me.

Matthew's comment here on training feels very fitting with the PP roles and ways of working.

Supporting Trainee Wellbeing

Across any of the training routes or roles, training courses will incorporate a variety of support mechanisms for trainees, with the recognition that there is a lot to complete within a short period of time and that trainee wellbeing is an important consideration in the process.

Some courses may include a question at the interview stage of recruitment, asking about self-care mechanisms or how potential trainees will manage the more challenging aspects of the course. This highlights the importance of proactively supporting wellbeing early on, so that the need for this doesn't come as a surprise further down the line.

These courses are accessed by adult learners who are completing the programme at a later point across the lifespan than young adults heading to university for the first time to undertake an undergraduate degree. Often, but not always, trainees on these programmes will already have an undergraduate degree and be returning to study. Others may have been in the workplace previously and are coming to these programmes with appropriate experience under their belt.

What we know about adult learners, that is particularly appropriate to the topic of supporting trainee wellbeing, is that adult learners often have many facets of life to balance alongside their studies. This may include (but not be limited to) partners, children, other caring responsibilities, their own interests, hobbies, or wider activities, as well as friendships, and potentially other financial considerations, or others who are financially dependent upon them.

Completing a PP training course may, in the short term, involve a reduction in pay for some, in particular if it is as part of a career change. Although, as many of us may say, "the money isn't everything", and certainly in the caring and healthcare professions isn't generally the first reason that people are drawn to the jobs, it should be acknowledged as a factor to be considered by trainees undertaking these types of courses and potentially any financial hardship can have an impact on overall wellbeing during an intense year of training.

All the factors above, alongside the nature of PP roles including high caseloads and work that can be emotive, can impact on wellbeing during the training year and beyond. Within the training year, there will be support available through a variety of sources including an allocated tutor on the programme, a wider team of lecturers and tutors, any relevant education provider support channels, service-based support and occupational health teams, and direct line managers and clinical supervisors.

It is good to see that, in recent years, there has been research focused on the wellbeing of PPs, including during training. Some of this was presented at the 2024 British Association of Behavioural and Cognitive Psychotherapies Annual Conference Low-Intensity Event (a featured event within the wider conference, specifically for us PPs!) and begins to include actions for training providers, services, supervisors, and practitioners themselves to take to make sure the training year is the best it can be, and leads to an enjoyable and rewarding career beyond.

It's great to see this focus on wellbeing in place, to ensure that training experiences are as good as they can be in this wonderfully rewarding training year, which we hope you have now learned much more about.

Box 8.1 References and wider reading

Health Education England. (2023). *Module aims and content of education mental health practitioner for children and young people curriculum (EMHP)*. Health Education England.

Health Education England. (2023). *Module aims and content of wellbeing practitioner for children and young people curriculum (CWP). V.3.* Health Education England.

NHS England. (2023). *National curriculum for psychological wellbeing practitioner (PWP) programmes. V.4.3.* NHS England.

NHS England. (2023). *National curriculum for mental health and wellbeing practitioners.* NHS England.

Chapter 9

Professional Ethics

Many roles within the fields of public service, and more specifically, health care, have requirements to abide by specified sets of professional ethics. This can be described in several ways, such as 'The Standards of Conduct, Performance, and Ethics' by the British Association of Behavioural and Cognitive Psychotherapies (BABCP) and the Health and Care Professions Council, or 'The Code' by the Nursing and Midwifery Council. Doctors in the United Kingdom are registered with the General Medical Council and must abide by their professional standards described as 'Good Medical Practice'.

In many cases, organisations will have one document that incorporates both general professional standards and guidance on the scope of the role and how safe, good-quality practice can be maintained, as well as consideration of ethical working within the role and how dilemmas, challenges, and breaches of professionalism will be handled. There are some cases where this guidance is split across multiple documents, and registrants should be aware of this when they are signing up.

It goes (hopefully) without saying that, in any of the professional roles that require registration and adherence to a practice code of conduct and ethics (however this is worded), the individual practitioner should be fully aware of the content of these documents to ensure that their practice is in line.

Registration for Psychological Wellbeing Practitioners (PWPs), Mental Health Wellbeing Practitioners (MHWPs), Children's Wellbeing Practitioners (CWPs), and Education Mental Health Practitioners (EMHPs) is currently available via two organisations – the

DOI: 10.4324/9781003542049-9

British Association of Behavioural and Cognitive Psychotherapy (BABCP) and the British Psychological Society (BPS). Two other roles, Clinical Associate in Psychology (CAP) and Clinical Associate in Applied Psychology (CAAP) are also eligible to apply specifically to the BPS Wider Psychological Workforce register (see Chapter 14 for more details on these).

For the BABCP, the register is called the Wellbeing Practitioner Register, whilst as previously mentioned the BPS register is called the Wider Psychological Workforce Register. Both registers are accredited by the Professional Standards Authority (PSA). This means that the organisations have satisfied the PSA's standards for how the registers are governed and managed, how complaints are handled, and that the standards registrants are asked to meet are appropriate.

Registration was initially launched for the PWP role in July 2021, becoming mandated by the National Health Service (NHS) England from June 2022. It took a little while longer for registration of CWPs and EMHPs to launch. This launch happened in April 2023, becoming an NHS England requirement from April 2024, in most cases as a condition of employment under the specified job title. Registration for MHWPs launched in June 2025.

As mentioned above, there are two organisations offering registration for PPs, the BABCP and the BPS. This setup, of having a choice of registering organisation, is not commonly seen. However, both organisations have clear links to the role and clear ways in which they can support the ongoing career progression of PPs, making sense of this unique arrangement. For example, we know that whilst the PP roles make rewarding careers in and of themselves, it is common for PPs to move on to other forms of training further into their careers. Some of the most frequent pathways taken are training in high-intensity cognitive behavioural therapy (CBT), which aligns to ongoing registration and membership with the BABCP, or doctoral-level training in psychology, which aligns to ongoing registration and membership with the BPS.

Whichever organisation a PP may choose for their registration, the underpinning criteria to be met to register are the same across both options, with some role-specific variation only. This chapter will continue and cover these criteria in summary; however, it is important to note that details should be checked with the registering organisations at the time at which you wish to register to ensure that you are working from the most up-to-date information.

Cross-Role Criteria

Some of the criteria to be met are consistent across all the PP roles, and we shall summarise these first, before moving on to the role-specific differences.

All PP roles registrants are required to:

- Be a member of the body with which you are registering.
  The BABCP has a standard membership, whereas the BPS has three different membership options. BPS offers graduate membership for those with a BPS-accredited undergraduate degree or BPS-accredited conversion course, full membership for a range of professionals using psychology in their job roles (see BPS website for details), and associate membership for those who are appropriate to join the Wider Psychological Workforce Register but do not meet the requirements for graduate or full membership.
- Have completed a BPS-accredited training programme.
  Although registration is offered via the BPS and the BABCP, it is important to note that course accreditation is only offered by the BPS. Even if you wish to register with the BABCP as a PP, the course you have completed will need to be accredited with the BPS (but don't worry, the courses deal with this – it isn't a job for you!).

  Because some courses existed before registration was launched for the role, there are alternative ways of recognising this. These are detailed in the role-specific sections of this chapter.
- Be in current employment in the specified system of care for the role.
  You can only apply for registration whilst you are in current employment in the relevant role. If you are having a break from practice, for example, as a career break or for parental leave, then there are options to maintain your registration if you are already registered (details of this further on in the chapter). However, you must be employed in the role at the time you are applying for registration. If you are not in current employment,

you would need to wait until you return to employment as a PP to apply for registration.

- Meet the minimum clinical practice requirements.
  There are some role-specific requirements about the type of practice being undertaken; however, the cross-role minimum requirement is two hours per week of clinical practice. It is further specified that this must include a mix of assessment and treatment work and must be 'live'. 'Live' work can include face to face, telephone, and video working, but cannot include computerised CBT where you are not interacting with the client or YP at the time.

- Be receiving supervision from an appropriately qualified supervisor.
  Supervisors must have completed or be in the process of completing appropriate training or meet the criteria for previous experience in supervising the PP role. The required training varies slightly across the roles.
  All supervisors should have appropriate levels of knowledge, skill, and experience in delivering low-intensity CBT interventions.

- Meet the minimum supervision requirements.
  You must be having clinical supervision at the specified minimum frequency and for a specified minimum duration to register. This is applicable to both types of supervision, as detailed below:

Clinical Case Management Supervision (CCMS)

This type of clinical supervision is focused on reviewing the caseload of the trainee PP. There is a clear structure around the order in which cases are presented and the level of detail that should be covered. This allows the supervisor to ensure the trainee is holding a suitably sized caseload, with the appropriate types of cases, and that the interventions being offered are in line with the remit of the role and the training that the trainee has received.

Clinical Skills Supervision* (CSS)

This type of clinical supervision is focused on developing the skills of the trainee PP. This can be done through a variety of methods such as watching recordings of clinical practice for the purpose of reflection, practicing skills through role-play or other activities, and discussion. CSS is generally provided in a group format, allowing trainees to learn from one another and engage in skills practice activities with peers as well as the supervisor.

*It should be noted that, for MHWPs, CSS is often referred to as psychological intervention supervision (PIS), including in the NHS role-specific guidance document "Mental Health Wellbeing Practitioner: A Guide to Practice". The format of PIS is broadly similar to CSS; however, some specific elements of MHWP supervision are covered in more detail in the role-specific chapter of this book (see Chapter 3 – Being a Mental Health Wellbeing Practitioner).

Supervision across the roles must also include live assessment of practice, which means that the supervisor must be able to see a video or audio recording of your practice or be able to join your session for live observation.

- Have paid your application and registration fees.
  This is the less popular criteria to meet; however, in line with many other registered professions in the world of health care, there is a cost to registration. The precise amount should be checked with the organisation you are registering with at the time of registration. It will usually include a one-time fee for applying and then a registration amount that will be charged annually.

  The fees have been set considering the standard rates of pay for PP roles, so they are less than some other psychological profession registration or accreditation costs.
- Work in line with the registering organisation's code of conduct.
  We began this chapter noting that many professions have codes of conduct by which they must abide, and the PP roles are no different. The precise code you will sign up to abide by will depend on the organisation with which you register. For the BPS, registrants must abide by the Member Conduct Rules, Code of Ethics and Conduct, and Fitness to Practice Framework. For the BABCP, it is the Standard of Conduct, Performance, and Ethics.

Role-Specific Criteria

Tables 9.1–9.4 cover role-specific variations and criteria. As noted above, details should be checked with the registering organisations at the time at which you wish to register to ensure that you are working from the most up-to-date information.

If the registration criteria are met and your PP registration is approved, you are then listed on the relevant public register. The information that is included on the register is slightly different across the two organisations. The BABCP lists your name, your unique BABCP membership number, the region in which you are working, and the status of your registration (e.g., registered). The BPS lists your name, the type of BPS membership you hold (e.g., graduate, full, or associate membership), the area in which you work, and your unique registration number. By clicking on the BPS register entry, it is also possible to see your full work address as the registrant, your language, and if any sanctions are held against you or not.

Table 9.1 PWP-specific registration criteria

PWP	
Training requirements	Where qualifying via an apprenticeship route, you must have completed the end-point assessment and have the apprenticeship certificate to evidence this.
	The only exception to completing an accredited PWP course is completion of the forerunner trainings, or the Health Education England (HEE) commissioned 2021 'PWP Assessment of Competence Scheme' which are both outlined in the NHS Talking Therapies Manual.
Practice requirements	The specified system of care for a PWP is a stepped-care pathway, such as an NHS Talking Therapies service, for adults.
	You must have six months of experience working in the specified system of care, which can include time as a trainee.
Supervision requirements	You must be receiving a minimum of one hour per week of CCMS and one hour per fortnight of CSS.
	All CSS supervisors must have completed or be in the process of completing specific NHS TT supervision training.

Table 9.2 CWP-specific registration criteria

CWP	
Training requirements	Where qualifying pre-2023, you must have completed a HEE Quality Assured CWP training programme (a list of these is available). If qualifying post-2023, the course should be BPS accredited.
Practice requirements	The specified system of care for a CWP is a stepped-care pathway supporting YP primarily 5–18 years old (and in all cases under 26 years old), usually employed by a CYPMH service. Any work undertaken with adults should focus on their role as parent or carer of the YP primarily being supported.
Supervision requirements	You must be receiving a minimum of one hour per fortnight of CCMS. For the first six months post-qualifying, you should receive a minimum of one hour per fortnight of CSS, which can be reduced to one hour per month after six months. All CSS supervisors must have completed or be in the process of completing specific CWP supervision training, or the SWP training programme, or have been providing supervision to CWPs (or EMHPs) for at least two years.

Table 9.3 EMHP-specific registration criteria

EMHP	
Training requirements	Where qualifying pre-2023, you must have completed a HEE Quality Assured EMHP training programme (a list of these is available). If qualifying post-2023, the course should be BPS accredited.
Practice requirements	The specified system of care for an EMHP is a Mental Health Support Team. Any work undertaken with adults should focus on their role as parent or carer of the YP primarily being supported.
Supervision requirements	You must be receiving a minimum of one hour per fortnight of CCMS. For the first six months post-qualifying, you should receive a minimum of one hour per fortnight of CSS, which can be reduced to one hour per month after six months. All CSS supervisors must have completed or be in the process of completing specific EMHP supervision training, or the SWP training programme, or have been providing supervision to EMHPs for at least two years.

Table 9.4 MHWP-specific registration criteria

MHWP	
Training requirements	The only exception to completing an accredited MHWP course is completion of one of two specific predecessor courses (University of Sussex Graduate Mental Health Practitioner and University of Central Lancashire Associate Psychological Practitioner – APP) where you have also undertaken the certificated HEE/NHS England approved conversion programme (at Sussex University, University of Central Lancashire, or Edge Hill University).
Practice requirements	The specified system of care for an MHWP is to be working in NHS-commissioned services for adults with severe mental health difficulties, where seamless access (no additional referral required) to additional support from an appropriate registered mental health professional is available if required. Acknowledging the element of care-planning within the MHWP role, you must spend a minimum of 50% of your time on psychological assessment, formulation, and interventions from the MHWP National Curriculum.
Supervision requirements	You must be receiving a minimum of one hour per week of CCMS and one hour per week of CSS. All CSS supervisors must have completed or be in the process of completing specific MHWP supervision training.

It should be noted that where there might be concerns around practitioner safety due to name and work location appearing on the register (e.g., in cases of stalking or domestic abuse), the BPS will look at cases on an individual basis and may be able to still register you as a PP and not display your details on the public register. The BABCP register lists your geographical region (e.g., North West, South East, etc.) and is therefore less specific about work location, which may mitigate concerns.

The registers for both the BABCP and BPS can be searched, via the organisation's website, by any member of the public. This can offer a level of assurance to the public if they are accessing or seeking support from a PP that the person has had sufficient training, is being sufficiently supervised, is undertaking sufficient continuing professional development (CPD) activity, and is abiding to the ethical practice guidance.

The structure and requirements set around training, practice, and supervision are also of benefit to you as a PP. They support you in ensuring that your job plan and working week include the elements required, and that you are not being used in ways that are outside the remit of your role or the reach of your training.

Katie Jamieson is a qualified CWP and current trainee Senior Wellbeing Practitioner (SWP). She tells us how much she values registration as a PP, saying, "Registration is great in terms of acknowledging the PP roles. It gets the roles out there as being legitimate routes for training and qualification and recognises the value PP roles bring to services".

Maintaining Registration

Registration as a PP is valid for one year and must be renewed annually. This involves making a declaration that you are still in current employment and working in the specified system of care relevant to your role, still receiving the appropriate level of supervision, and continuing to abide by the ethical codes for your registering organisation.

Within your declaration, you must also confirm that you have completed the required amount of CPD activity across the previous 12 months. There are slight variations in the specific CPD requirements across the two registering bodies, which should be checked at the time of registering.

However, generally, it is around five activities across the year, with some of these needing to directly relate to CBT-informed approaches or other role-specific ways of working, for example, CPD underpinned by social learning theory for CWPs and EMHPs, or CPD linked to whole school approaches for EMHPs specifically.

Gaps in Registration and Leaving the Role

As mentioned earlier, it is possible to have a break in practice and then return to a registered PP role. If the break is temporary and less than two years, the registering organisation can be advised of this and your registration can continue so long as appropriate fees are still paid.

If registration and membership fees are not continued, then your registration will lapse, and you will no longer appear on the register. The registration will need to be reinstated, and fees paid for you to be shown on the register again.

If the break in practice is longer than two years, you will be required to re-apply for registration (with additional application fees applied) and may be required to provide additional information to support this return to practice. Further details can be found via the registering organisations.

If you leave the PP role and are no longer working within the scope of PP practice or the specified system of care, then you must inform the registering body of this and resign from the register.

There are some other changes that you must also inform your registering body of, including a change of employer or a change of supervisor, as well as your general details (name, address, contact email, etc.).

Conclusion

The benefits of registration and working within a framework that supports ethical working and accountability for practice have hopefully come across in this chapter. Registration of the PP roles was something that initially PWPs (the elder sibling in the PP family) began to push for, and the fact that it is now in place for PWPs, CWPs, EMHPs, and, most recently, MHWPs is a huge achievement and milestone for PPs.

However, it would be remiss to wrap up this chapter without noting that PPs have been working effectively and in an appropriately ethical way since the roles were initially rolled out. PPs have always been taught to work within the scope of their training, making use of evidence-based interventions, and in a way that is collaborative and person-centred. They have always been supervised robustly and utilised measurement (whether you call these minimum data set (MDS), routine outcome measures (ROMs), or patient reported outcome measures (PROMs) to demonstrate accountability.

It isn't that registration has produced ethical low-intensity working, but what it has done is to ensure that this is consistently applied across all roles, regions, and services. It has put a framework around the roles that also gives recognition and protection. And that can only be a good thing.

Box 9.1 References and wider reading

Health Education England. (2023). *Module aims and content of education mental health practitioner for children and young people curriculum (EMHP).* Health Education England.

Health Education England. (2023). *Module aims and content of wellbeing practitioner for children and young people curriculum (CWP). V.3.* Health Education England.

NHS England. (2023). *National curriculum for psychological wellbeing practitioner (PWP) programmes. V.4.3.* NHS England.

NHS England. (2023). *National curriculum for mental health and wellbeing practitioners.* NHS England.

Chapter 10

Mastering the Job Market

Some of our previous chapters have been written based upon, and summarising, the documents and publications that underpin the psychological practitioner (PP) roles, including guidance from National Health Service (NHS) England, national curriculums for PP training courses, and information disseminated by the registering bodies, British Psychological Society (BPS) and the British Association for Behavioural and Cognitive Psychotherapies (BABCP).

This chapter by its very nature has had to be written a little bit differently, as there isn't specific guidance out there on how to master the job market as a Psychological Wellbeing Practitioner (PWP), Mental Health Wellbeing Practitioner (MHWP), Children's Wellbeing Practitioner (CWP), or Education Mental Health Practitioner (EMHP). We couldn't draw upon a published document that guides newly qualified trainees, or experienced practitioners ready for a change, on what to do. Instead, what we have aimed for in this chapter is to include the voices, opinions, and ideas from a range of people involved in the process of employing PPs.

We hope that this will offer a range of hints, tips, and ideas to those looking to find employment, covering the different PP roles and applicable to the range of services and geographic regions you may be looking to work within.

This is all the while considering that on completion of PP training, in whichever of the roles, there is, of course, the hope that the service within which you have worked as a trainee will be able to offer you a qualified role to continue within. This is the ideal outcome, not only for employment security, and subsequently

DOI: 10.4324/9781003542049-10

trainee wellbeing, as you move into the final months of training, but also for continuity as a practitioner. Staying within a service that is familiar, with familiar systems, processes, and continuity of supervision, will support practitioners at a time where there is a stepping away from teaching days. Caseloads will likely increase to fill the days that were previously protected teaching time.

Does this mean that practitioners who are not able to continue in the service they trained within should be worried? No, not at all. So long as the requirements of the training year are completed before moving on from the training service placement, and the new service is an appropriate system of care for the role (more detail on this further into this chapter), able to support the qualified practitioner in meeting the requirements of registration, then moving services is not necessarily problematic.

However, what it does mean is that there may be some additional considerations needed. If the move into a qualified role is also accompanied by a move to a new service, with new systems, processes, colleagues, and supervisors, then this just also needs holding in mind.

The types of things, in particular, that may be useful to acknowledge and think about if moving to a new service could include the following:

- What goals for supervision were in place during the training year? Were these met? Do they need adjusting and/or carrying over to your new supervisor?
- What standard elements of practice specific to the role might the training year have given less opportunity for you to develop skills and confidence in?

    For example, as an EMHP did the training year give sufficient opportunity to develop whole school approach (WSA) skills or is this an area that would benefit from focus in your first year of qualification?

    For a PWP, this may be a specific intervention that there has been less opportunity to practice. For a CWP, it may be delivering staff training. Or for an MHWP, it may be case management approaches. Really, any element of the role can come up more or less frequently during the training year, leaving opportunity for you to focus and hone skills once qualified.

Looking for PP Roles

When it comes to looking for a new opportunity for a PP role, or your first opportunity for a qualified role post-training, much of our advice will be similar to that given for looking for an initial trainee post in Chapter 6 – Routes into the Profession (see Chapter 6 for further details).

A great place to begin is the NHS jobs website (www.jobs.nhs. uk). This is where jobs within NHS trusts are advertised, and this covers many of the PP roles. The best terms to search for when trying to identify roles will be the words contained in the job titles themselves. It is worth remembering that there may be some slight regional differences in job titles.

As well as the NHS, there are some other types of organisations, such as mental health charities, that may employ PPs (depending on the specific role, PWP, MHWP, CWP, or EMHP). These organisations sometimes form part of local mental health partnership offers.

As mentioned in our earlier chapter in relation to seeking trainee roles (Chapter 6 – Routes into the Profession), knowing the types of mental health service providers and the local offer in the areas you are looking to work in can also give you additional places to search for advertised roles. Organisations may advertise any available roles on their own websites, via any social media platforms they use, or via more generalised job websites. As with the NHS jobs website, searching for words and terms related to the job titles can bring up appropriate results.

When you are reviewing job adverts, it is important to check that the job is the right fit for you, as a PWP, CWP, EMHP, or MHWP. This might include checking that the role offers access to the right types of cases, in the right system of care, with the right type of supervision and support available. Although there are some similarities across the PP roles, as the role-specific chapters in this book have demonstrated, there are key differences too (see Chapters 2–5 for further details).

It would not be a good use of your time or energy to complete an application form and potentially attend an interview for a role that, turns out, isn't able to employ you in a way that supports your ongoing registration. As a reminder, the specified systems of care for each role are detailed in Table 10.1.

Table 10.1 Specified systems of care

Role	Specified System of Care
PWP	Be working in a stepped-care pathway, such as an NHS Talking Therapies service, for adults.
MHWP	Be working in NHS-commissioned services for adults with severe mental health difficulties, where seamless access (no additional referral required) to additional support from an appropriate registered mental health professional is available if required.
CWP	Be working within a stepped-care pathway supporting YP primarily 5–18 years old (and in all cases under 26 years old), usually employed by a CYPMH service.
EMHP	Be working within an MHST.

Further information on what the requirements are to acquire and maintain registration in your role can be found on the BPS and BABCP websites.

What Are Employers Looking For?

There are some skills, attributes, and qualities that will be desirable to employees of PPs whether it is a training post or a qualified position. Some of these are summarised in our earlier chapter on Routes into the Profession (see Chapter 6), as well as being considered in the chapter on transferable skills (see Chapter 7). They might include, but not be limited to, organisation and time management skills, qualities of resilience and adaptability, skills in creativity, or the ability to communicate effectively with people of all ages.

There are also some things that employers may be looking for and wanting to see demonstrated across applications, personal statements, and interviews, which are likely to be more specific to qualified positions. These may be helpful to consider if you are moving on from a training post at the end of your training year, or if you are looking for a qualified PP role at any stage in your career.

These more specific elements might include, again without being limited to, experience of delivering the full range of interventions offered in the relevant PP role or evidence of relevant continued professional development whilst working in the role.

Sara Yunus, a Service Lead for a Mental Health Support Team (MHST, where EMHPs are based), says that on top of the skills and attributes that would be wanted in a trainee, in a qualified practitioner she would be looking for "a good working knowledge of risk assessment and management, and awareness of how to manage any presenting safeguarding issues".

If you are applying for a qualified position at a further point in your career, rather than at the end of your training year, then the new employer may want to know that you have previously obtained registration and will be able to maintain this in your new role.

Applications and Personal Statements

It may sound obvious, but one of the first bits of advice that can be given in relation to reviewing job advertisements and completing application forms is to ensure that you read everything through thoroughly. Maybe even read things through a couple of times, to ensure that you are clear on what they are looking for, and on what criteria are essential or desirable for the post.

These criteria are usually included in the job description, or an additional document called a person specification, where they might be split into lists of essential or desirable criteria, or listed within a table with columns that indicate along the side whether the criteria are essential or desirable.

These columns may also indicate where the employer expects you to demonstrate that you can meet these criteria, for example, via the application form (sometimes indicated as 'A'), via references, via document or certificate checks, or via interview (sometimes indicated as 'I').

Now that you are a qualified PP, it is likely that the requirements will include, as mentioned above, acquiring or maintaining registration in the relevant role. Therefore, it is recommended to note your registration on the application, either in the specified place or if there isn't one, by mentioning it in your statement.

When completing your application form, it is important to make sure that you identify how you meet all the essential criteria. Some of these may be covered by the details you are required to fill in, such as your qualifications, previous employment, and so on. Other essential criteria might need to be included in a personal statement, explaining how you meet them. For example, if you are asked to demonstrate an ability to deliver low-intensity cognitive behavioural therapy (CBT) interventions effectively, then this would be necessary to expand on in a personal or supporting statement. This not only demonstrates that you know what these interventions are but also that you know how to check if your work is effective. Evidence of effectiveness might include reference to outcomes of cases (anonymised of course), or feedback you have received on your work.

It is also important to include information on how you meet as many of the desirable criteria as you can. PP posts can be competitive, so ensuring that you show how you can meet these additional, desirable qualities and skills will give you a better chance of being shortlisted to make it to the interview stage.

These final bits of advice may sound obvious but are likely still worth saying and bearing in mind when completing application forms. Checking spelling is important, so that your application looks as professional as possible. If the application system you are using is online and doesn't have the spellcheck facility included, it can be useful to write out any supporting statements (or longer blocks of text) in a Word document first so that you can spell check it there. You can then usually copy and paste this back into the online application form.

Getting someone else to read through your application and any required supporting statement can also spot any spelling mistakes, and check that it reads clearly and coherently. It doesn't necessarily matter whether the person who is reading it for you is knowledgeable about the roles, or this field of work, as the focus of reading through is about checking how clear it is. They may also be able to check against the essential and desirable criteria for you, to ensure that you have mentioned how you meet them.

Interviews

When you are offered an interview for a qualified post, what might you need to consider or do to prepare? You will have completed at least one interview in relation to PP working already, to get onto your training course. Will this interview experience for a qualified role differ? We would say yes *and* no, there are some things that will be similar; however, there are also some key differences.

One of the things that will likely be the same might be the broad structure and setup of the interview. Many services utilise experts-by-experience, meaning those who have lived (which generally refers to historic, or previous) experience and/or living (referring to current or ongoing) experience of mental health difficulties and using the service previously, are included as members of the interview panels.

As qualified practitioners will likely know, inclusion of lived experience within recruitment is very much in line with the ethos and principles of the NHS Talking Therapies for Anxiety and Depression (formerly Improving Access to Psychological Therapies or IAPT) and Children and Young People's Psychological Trainings (CYP PT – formerly Children and Young People's Improving Access to Psychological Therapies or CYP IAPT) programmes. Within CYP PT, this also links into the principle of 'participation' (see Chapters 4 and 5, on being a CWP or EMHP for further details on these principles) and is included as one of the nine participation priorities, with priority number 5 being 'involve young people in recruitment'.

As with your trainee position interview, we would reiterate for your qualified interview that it is important to remember to be punctual, be this turning up on time at a location or joining an online meeting promptly, to give a good first impression. If travelling somewhere in person, check your route and any public transport or parking requirements as needed. If joining an interview remotely, make sure that you have the right link or code to hand in plenty of time.

Although PP roles can involve working in community settings, or with children and young people, which may require adopting a less formal approach to support engagement, it is still important to remember to convey professionalism during the interview and associated interactions. Professionalism can be demonstrated through choice of clothing, manner, language, and wider communication (verbal, non-verbal, and written), as well as via the content you refer to.

Although interviewers will want to get a sense of your personality as an individual, they will be looking for someone who can represent their organisation well during the training year (both in practice and when on training days) and beyond. As a qualified practitioner, you will likely have the advantage of being aware of professional standards expected through your experience of the training year, registration requirements, and working beyond your training. Ensuring this is demonstrated in your interview is a good idea.

Because you will have specific PP experience to draw on in your interview, we would say that it is more important than ever to include examples of this in relation to all questions you are asked. Making links to practice shows that you are a 'working practitioner', rather than having just a theoretical understanding of the job.

Sara Yunus (who we met earlier in the chapter) backs this up, saying that, ideally in an interview, she would want a potential employee to be able to talk through examples from their practice to thoroughly demonstrate their understanding. As previously mentioned, Sara would expect qualified applicants to have good knowledge of risk assessment and management, and including an example from practice to demonstrate this would fit with the importance of risk assessment.

Even though PPs are designed to work with those who have minimal to no presenting risk, the ability to effectively assess for this and manage anything that is disclosed or uncovered is a top priority. Where someone applying for a trainee position may have the opportunity to develop their skills in this area across the training year, for a qualified position employers, like Sara, are looking for someone with a fuller working knowledge and level of experience.

As well as being able to talk through an example of managing risk, talking through examples of where qualified practitioners have delivered low-intensity CBT interventions is something that Sara would like to see in an interview. Sara says,

> If a candidate at interview can talk us through an example of a case they have completed, telling us for example how change was monitored and what the intervention consisted of, then this demonstrates their working knowledge of the role really well.

Marianne Tay, Course Lead for an MHWP programme and experienced CBT therapist, shares similar thoughts. She says,

> The interview is all about demonstrating what you say you can do, and in every answer, you should give the panel an

explanation of when you have previously evidenced your abilities. Remember, it is far better to be talking too much in an interview than too little. Do not assume that your application and curriculum vitae (CV) will speak for themselves, you need to be able to communicate what you can do. The main thing you can bring to an interview is passion for the role, and for the organisation that you are interviewing with!

Melissa Street, a consultant psychological therapist and former CWP Programme Lead, says similar, telling us,

> Think about how you've developed and gained experience, in your career in general but also across your training year and since qualifying. Where you can, make links from this to what is being asked for the in PP job role. That will stand out to interviewers and recruiters.

Paul Thompson, a qualified PWP, senior lecturer in mental health, and Director of the Psychological Professionals' Development Hub, tells us,

> One thing that's important to understand is that the PWP role is not just a stepping stone, it is a profession in its own right, with a clearly defined scope of practice and has a vital place within the stepped-care model.

Matthew Beaton is a principal mental health practitioner and honorary lecturer on an MHWP programme and highlights the same point. He says,

> I would avoid referring to the role as a 'stepping stone'. While you may have future ambitions, such as becoming a High-Intensity Therapist or a Clinical Psychologist, it's important to respect the MHWP role as a valuable and meaningful career.

Paul and Matthew make an important point, and one that it is useful to hold in mind when applying for qualified training posts. Although, as we've already noted, employers will likely want to hear that practitioners are open to developing their skills and potentially undertaking further training, it is important to also show dedication to the role itself, and appreciation for it as a valid career.

The idea of the PP roles being 'stepping stones' on to 'bigger and better things*' was certainly prevalent in the early days of the roles, and this way of thinking may not have entirely gone away yet, although there has definitely been a shift in the landscape (*not that either author believes other modalities or roles to be bigger or better, remaining practitioners themselves, but we hope that this phrase conveys the idea).

Paul sums up well the balance that needs to be struck, telling us,

PP roles open doors to a range of career pathways in mental health but do not be in a rush to move on quickly. You will need time to embed your clinical skills and consolidate your learning. For people who are reflective, values-driven, and open to feedback, the role offers significant opportunities for personal and professional growth.

If you are able to demonstrate, within an interview process, your desire to continue and develop in a practitioner role either as a long-term career or to ensure that you have embedded those valuable skills before moving on to a different role or training, then this will likely put you in a favourable position with the panel. We wish you the best of luck!

Box 10.1 References and wider reading

British Association of Behavioural and Cognitive Psychotherapies (BABCP) website – https://babcp.com/

British Psychological Society (BPS) website – https://www.bps.org.uk/

NHS Jobs website – www.jobs.nhs.uk

Chapter 11

Starting Out

Introduction

Congratulations! You've completed your training and are now a qualified psychological practitioner (PP); take time to acknowledge this achievement. It is acknowledged elsewhere in this book that the training year can be tough, so you should be rightly proud of demonstrating and achieving the competencies required to become a qualified PP.

However, it is also important to realise that your learning and development does not stop here. To be the best practitioner, you can be requires a commitment to ongoing learning and development that is as long as your career, to ensure you are providing your clients with the best quality and up-to-date care.

The focus of this chapter will be on the first year of post-qualification for each of the PP roles, considering how the learning from the training year can be further embedded and built upon, what the transition can include, and how experience will broaden in this period.

There will be information about the role of supervision in this year, including an overview of the changing frequency (as outlined by registering bodies). Goal setting will be discussed in relation to identifying gaps in experience and having clear objectives for development, with an acknowledgement that there is a continuing process of learning and development through this first year – both in clinical confidence and skills such as caseload management.

This chapter will make use of case studies, with experienced practitioners from across the roles answering the question 'What did your first year as a qualified PP look, and feel, like?'

DOI: 10.4324/9781003542049-11

Registration

On qualification, PP roles are subject to registration. This registration is your responsibility as an individual practitioner, is a recommended contract requirement for provider services, and, amongst the many benefits, helps us provide assurance to our clients; therefore, it should be one of your very first jobs as a qualified practitioner.

There are two bodies that hold Wellbeing Practitioner Registers – The British Psychological Society (BPS) and the British Association for Behavioural and Cognitive Psychotherapies (BABCP). They provide equivalent offers for practitioners.

The BPS accredits the practitioner courses, but individual practitioners can register with either the BPS or the BABCP. The full background and rationale to practitioner registration can be found in Chapter 9.

The choice of which body (BPS or BABCP) to register with is down to personal preference, potential considerations could include previous background or future aspirations. Full details on the benefits and processes of registering are available on the two organisations' websites. Once eligible for registration, take time to consider the information provided by both the BPS and BABCP to help you make an informed decision on which organisation suits your individual needs best.

For both the BPS and BABCP, you first need to become a member of that organisation, but this can be done at the same time as registering as a practitioner, if you are not already an existing member of one.

In addition to being a member, you need to have completed the relevant accredited practitioner course, be able to provide your transcript, and complete the application form. You will be confirming you are working in an appropriate system of care and to your role-specific competencies and in accordance with the Fitness to Practise Framework (BPS) or Standards of Conduct, Performance, and Ethics (BABCP).

You will also need to ask your current clinical skills supervisor to complete a Supervisor's Report (BABCP) or a Clinical Skills Supervisor Confirmation Form (BPS). They will need to be practicing clinically themselves and have been supervising your practice for a minimum of six months. If they have been supervising you for less than six months, you will be required to provide additional evidence, as listed on the BABCP/BPS websites.

You can apply once you have six months of clinical practice experience; usually, this will be achieved as you reach the end of your training year.

Once you have gained your initial registration, you then need to maintain it. You do this by completing an 'Annual Declaration' and paying your fees (membership and registration) to your chosen body (BPS or BABCP). The declaration checks that you remain working in a specified system of care, are receiving the correct amounts of case management and clinical skills supervision (CSS) (see the table below) from an appropriately qualified supervisor, and are working within your specific role competencies.

In a year, you also need to complete your annual continuing professional development (CPD) hours. It is good practice to spread these throughout the year. The stipulation is that each year a practitioner will complete five learning and development activities, to include a minimum of six hours cognitive behavioural therapy (CBT)-informed skills development. In addition, the BPS clarifies the requirements for the specific practitioner roles as follows:

For PWPs, at least three out of the five activities they complete must directly relate to relevant CBT-informed approaches or CBT principles relating to core aspects of clinical activity. One of the activities and reflection should be on the clinical supervision you receive.

For CWPs, their CPD should be from relevant approaches underpinned by CBT and/or social learning theory. One of the activities and reflection should be on the clinical supervision you receive.

For EMHPs, their CPD should be from relevant approaches underpinned by CBT, social learning theory, and whole school approaches. One of the activities and reflection should be on the clinical supervision you receive.

For MHWPs, at least three of the five activities must directly relate to relevant CBT principles relating to core aspects of clinical activity undertaken. One of the activities and reflection should be on the clinical supervision you receive.

Table 11.1 Examples of suitable CPD evidence

CPD for Registration	
Example of CPD Activity	*Examples of Evidence*
In-service training	Course certificates
Journal Clubs	Course assignment feedback
Skills practice groups	Case studies
Lecturing/teaching	Guidance materials/guidelines
Service audits	Reflective statements

The practitioner must keep a log of reflective statements for each CPD activity completed; templates are available on the BABCP and BPS websites and any relevant certificates, and so on. You will need to provide this information if you are selected for a random audit. It should be noted that CPD requirements cannot be calculated pro rata, and the requirements are the same for full-time and part-time staff.

Table 11.1 shows some examples from the BABCP of CPD activities and the evidence that would be required to demonstrate completion. This is not an exhaustive summary, and a fuller list can be seen on the BABCP website.

In addition, you will also need to complete at least two observed practices, each year. Your supervisor should be able to observe you working with at least two clients, demonstrating at least two interventions, either live, through one-way screen or video or audio recording.

Observations support services to ensure good governance, for example, practitioners' adherence to low-intensity models and competent delivery of interventions; in addition, practitioners should see these observations of practice as an opportunity for further learning and development of their practice.

There is further information in Chapter 9 on professional ethics and standards of practice for PPs.

Changes to Supervision

Supervision is crucial to safe and effective practice and must continue once a practitioner is qualified; however, upon qualification,

Table 11.2 CMS and CSS requirements

	CWP	EMHP	PWP	MHWP
CMS	One hour per fortnight	One hour per fortnight	One hour per week	One hour per week
CSS	One hour per fortnight until six months post-qualified then one hour per month	One hour per fortnight until six months post-qualified then one hour per month	One hour per fortnight	One hour per fortnight

there are adjustments to levels of supervision to the following frequencies outlined in Table 11.2.

Your supervisor must also be appropriately qualified to deliver the supervision they offer.

Reality of the First Year

It has been a little while since the authors originally qualified, but even so, we remember the satisfaction of qualifying, tempered with the continued steep learning curve and adjustments to a qualified caseload in the first year.

Every newly qualified practitioner will have a unique journey and start to qualified life; however, below are the reflections of some practitioners who have qualified within the last few cohorts of their individual practitioner role, to give a flavour of the experiences the authors have most frequently encountered. The practitioners below were asked: 'What did your first year as a qualified PP look, and feel, like?'

Since qualifying, I have had such a diverse workload which keeps the role both engaging and fulfilling. The range of deliveries, from one-to-one sessions, to various group courses, has helped me build a wide range of skills. This variety has made me feel more capable in my role and has increased my confidence. I receive consistent support from my managers both within daily responsibilities and in pursuing any additional training in areas I am passionate about, such as perinatal mental health.

Madeleine Shimwell, Qualified PWP

My favourite thing about my role is seeing the gradual shifts in client's mental health. When something 'clicks', and they begin to feel more in control of their thoughts or behaviours, it makes the work feel meaningful. I also enjoy the structure of the role, especially the variety of interventions and sessions I get to deliver.

The most challenging aspect of my role is the high volume of clients, and the admin associated with each, especially when you're trying to balance this with maintaining the quality of interventions. It can be easy to feel stretched. I've quickly learned the importance of staying organised. Diary management, planning sessions, and having templates for various written documents has been a lifesaver. It's been a learning curve, but I feel I'm growing into the role and gaining confidence along the way.

I think that the PWP role is valuable because it offers accessible support to people who might otherwise face long waits or high thresholds to get help. Step 2 interventions are often the first introduction someone has to mental health treatment, so it's a privilege to be part of that early stage.

Vongai Tepa, Qualified PWP

As someone with no clinical experience prior to this role it has been a steep learning curve understanding how the organisational and business side of the NHS works and I still have a lot to learn about this. It's important to understand where the role fits, both within your own service and within the wider multi-disciplinary teams.

Adam Hope, Qualified MHWP

Since my late ADHD diagnosis and autism diagnosis, I feel that my neurodivergence helps my practice. Now in my early 50s, the hypervigilance developed from years of being undiagnosed allows me to keenly observe body language, facial expressions, and intonation, helping me detect subtle cues from young people (YP) during sessions. This sensitivity aids in identifying discomfort or unease, prompting timely interventions.

My experiences enable me to recognize challenges, especially in females, that might be overlooked in busy school environments. Through supervision discussions, I've collaborated with schools to gain necessary support.

Louise Rawley, Qualified EMHP

My first year was very much up and down. Initially I did not feel a sense of belonging. I was not getting any cases either, I wasn't sure if they knew my role. My supervisor emailed across different teams regarding cases and this is when I met a team that were amazing. They were so welcoming and accommodating. My first cases came from there and I still am working with them. With the course having new changes and us being the first cohort to experience these, it was difficult at times to manage the logistics of assignments within a community setting.

A lot happened in my personal life too. Workwise I was getting cases from across my local area, which meant I was travelling everywhere and that took its to. But, certain teams made it worth it and helped me want to stay and finish my qualification, which I am glad I did. It took me around 2 years in total to complete my qualification due to not being able to get certain cases to meet the portfolio requirements. Once done, I took a break. If it wasn't that, I would have left.

However, coming back, I was able to express my concerns and needs, which were accommodated for. I am now happy in my role and have developed many links within the community. I have been able to have freedom in pursuing the areas I want to work in e.g. ethnic diverse communities and have been fully supported. My supervisor has been amazing and this was another reason why I did not leave. I am very grateful for her.

Safa Asif, Qualified CWP

As Safa expresses in her reflection, the journey is not always easy or straightforward, but help and support are available, and finding your place with your role can lead to many positive experiences and development opportunities.

Ongoing Learning and Development

Even after many years of practice, one of the things that all psychological professionals will agree on is that learning and development do not stop. This is never truer than in a practitioner's first year post-qualification.

Your qualification means you have been passed as competent, but, in your first year, you will be required to increase your caseload to qualified levels, have to 'take from the top of the waiting list', and continue to meet clients who are all individuals! So, you may be competent, but you will need to continue to develop and hone your skills and grow in confidence.

Depending on your service, you may have access to a Preceptorship and/or a Professional Development Review or equivalent process. Often, this will run alongside your required case management supervision (CMS), CSS, and line management, with one or two named individuals for these checking in with you in the form of 'Review Meetings' exploring your learning, reflections, and progress over the course of your first qualified year.

Preceptorship

Preceptorship is defined as the period, to support a 'newly qualified practitioner' in, normally, their 'first year post-qualification'. It refers to support, plans, policy, programme, or documents designed to support the transition from trainee to fully functioning qualified team member. It is not about retesting your competency but supporting your continued growth, confidence, and wellbeing in the role.

The preceptee is the person undergoing the Preceptorship, and their preceptor is the named professional, more experienced in the role, of the same or a higher Agenda for Change Banding than the preceptee, supporting them.

Preceptorship is explicitly mentioned in the NHS Talking Therapies Manual (NHS England, 2024) and MHWP Curriculum (NHS England, 2023). The Psychological Professions Network provides guidance on PP Preceptorship for all practitioner roles. This guidance and its two associated documents (PPs Preceptorship Quick Reference Guide and PP CPD) are predominantly designed to support services in their development of preceptorship for their practitioners and advise on CPD requirements; however, it provides links to a range of background information and resources that may be of interest to those reading this book.

Whichever Preceptorship model and/or paperwork your service uses, and in conjunction with your CMS, CSS, and line management, goal setting is something that you can utilise to support yourself and your development in this first year (and beyond).

As preceptorship is not about testing competency, it is important to consider what you want to achieve.

In the high-volume, often fast-paced world of low-intensity practice, being confident in your clinical decision-making is important, and this may form the basis of an early goal. However, it is important to stress that this is not a case of 'knowing everything' and 'doing everything'. It is just as important to know when to signpost and when to seek supervision and support.

As you meet more clients and presentations, there may be particular interventions and how to apply these to specific cases that you feel you need to focus on. These may be interventions that you had less opportunity to utilise during your training year, or maybe there is an intervention you just feel less confident in. CMS may help you identify areas of focus for goals, and if these are skills or intervention-based, CSS may provide an opportunity to explore these further. Or if you identify a specific need, then you might find CPD helps you meet this goal.

And, of course, the goal we began this chapter with: to achieve Wellbeing Practitioner Registration!

So, supervision (CMS and CSS), line management, and self-reflection can help you to identify gaps in experience, but how can we use goal setting to support the development of clear objectives to advance your skills and practice?

Many practitioners, or those aspiring to the roles, will be aware of SMART Goals. A goal is defined as something which we set ourselves and work towards to achieve. It is a specific aim or target we wish to complete to help us overcome an identified problem. Initially coined by Doran (1981), a SMART goal stands for Specific, Measurable, Achievable, Relevant, and Time-bound.

When setting goals for ourselves, it is important to follow a few simple guidelines to make sure that the goals we give ourselves are achievable; all goals should be SMART:

Specific: You should clearly define the goal. It should deal with a specific, identified problem.

Manageable: You should be able to complete your goal – don't pick something too difficult (or too easy) to begin with. Build up your goals over time. Break a larger goal down into smaller manageable chunks if this helps.

Achievable: Pick a problem you can overcome. Achieving things will make you feel good, so go for something you can do, even if it is a little difficult.

Relevant: The goal should be personal and meaningful to you. If you can achieve your goal, how will life change for you? Will it change for the better?

Timed: You should set yourself a time in which to achieve your goal and keep to it. Having an indefinite time to complete the goal might mean you keep putting off achieving it!

Setting goals is not always easy, and to begin with, you may need help; this is fine. If you are an aspiring practitioner, perhaps ask a trusted friend or family member. If you are a trainee or have a contact within the psychological professions, you could see if they are able to provide some feedback. They may support you to come up with ideas you had not considered or be able to help you see whether your goals are too hard or too easy to begin with. You should, however, aim towards working on your goals by yourself.

You should review your goals regularly and monitor your progress. If you have broken down a goal into smaller chunks, remember to move on to the next one once you have achieved the first.

In Box 11.1 we have provided one composite clinical example and one hypothetical personal development example of goal setting to illustrate how this strategy can be applied both with clients but also to aid personal development:

Box 11.1 SMART goal examples

Practice Example Smart Goal – Clinical

Albert identifies that he has a problem with busy shops. He avoids shopping as he is worried he will get flustered and not be able to cope with all the packing and paying for goods (**Specific**). Albert's wife now does all their shopping despite the fact that she has very bad arthritis and finds it difficult to carry shopping bags. Albert wants to be able to help his wife and decides to set himself some goals.

Albert decides the problem is too big to deal with all in one go and decides to break it down (**Manageable**). He asks his wife to help him, and she agrees.

Albert's first goal is to go to the shops with his wife in the morning during the week (when it will be quiet) and stay for 30 minutes, and then buy 5 items from a list (**Achievable**). Albert will do this for 3 days (**Timed**).

Once he has achieved this, Albert decides on a second goal, he will go to the shops the same as before, on a week day morning, with a list and stay for 30 minutes, but without his wife.

Albert's final goal was to go to the shops on Saturday afternoon by himself, when it would be busy. He would take a shopping list and get all the items before he returned home.

Albert was now able to go to the shops for his wife, especially when she wasn't feeling well (**Relevant**).

Practice Example Smart Goal – Personal Development

Samira is a newly qualified PP. She has identified that she is finding the Behavioural Activation intervention more challenging to explain to her clients than any other intervention (**Specific**).

Samira has a Clinical Skills Session booked for the following week (**Timed**). Where she will have the support of her supervisor (**Manageable**).

Samira wants to be able to deliver interventions to her clients in adherence to the clinical model (**Relevant**) and to a high standard (this is not **Specific** – Samira should work to clarify what this means).

Samira can work with her Supervisor, using CSS to develop and practice her B/A explanation.

Samira can then implement the practiced skill with her client (**Achievable**).

Table 11.3 Space to consider setting your own goals

Goal	How will you know when you have achieved this goal?

This ability to reflect (covered in Chapter 7) and also apply interventions to self, as in the goal-setting example above, is also a technique used in training. It supports self-management of wellbeing (Chapter 12) but also helps to develop understanding and skill in delivering the interventions.

Take a moment now, using Table 11.3, to have a go at setting some of your own personal goals. These could be your next career steps or more personally driven:

There is plenty of evidence that SMART Goals can improve effectiveness and increase success, particularly when they are shared, which would suggest sharing and tracking them with your preceptor, trusted friend, family member, or colleague could be really beneficial in supporting you to achieve your own goals (Traugott, 2014).

Box 11.2 References and wider reading

BABCP Wellbeing Practitioner Registration. https://babcp.com/Wellbeing-Registrations/About

BPS Wider Psychological Workforce Register. https://www.bps.org.uk/wider-psychological-workforce

Doran, G.T. (1981). There's a S.M.A.R.T. way to write management's goals and objectives. *Management Review*, **70** (11), pp. 35–36.

NHS England. (2023). *National curriculum for mental health and wellbeing practitioners*. NHS England.

NHS England. (2024). *NHS talking therapies for anxiety and depression manual. 7th Edition*. NHS England. https://www.england.nhs.uk/wp-content/uploads/2018/06/nhs-talking-therapies-manual-v7.1-updated.pdf

Traugott, J. (2014). *Achieving your goals: An evidence-based approach*. Michigan State University. 2014–08–26. Retrieved 2024-01-09. Achieving your goals: An evidence-based approach - MSU Extension

Making the Most of Your Career

Introduction

In this chapter, we explore making the most of your career as a psychological practitioner (PP), following consolidating your skills and increasing your confidence in your first year post-qualification (Chapter 11).

Chapter 12 will explore the second year (and beyond!) Championing, the ways in which practitioners can grow in their roles. This will include connection to other practitioners via avenues such as the Psychological Professions Network (PPN) and special interest groups (SIGs), as well as making use of continuing professional development (CPD) to support ongoing development.

Ways to develop within the role will be explored, including further training and promotion opportunities such as becoming a supervisor, stepping into a senior role, or for Children's Wellbeing Practitioners (CWPs) and Educational Mental Health Practitioners (EMHPs) undertaking the Senior Wellbeing Practitioner (SWP) Postgraduate Diploma. We will also consider potential areas of specialism, such as training in working with long-term conditions (LTCs) for Psychological Wellbeing Practitioners (PWPs).

Elspeth and Kirsty want this chapter to demonstrate that the practitioner roles are satisfying destination careers in their own rights, roles to be proud of, grow and develop in.

Connecting with the Wider Practitioner Family

In your first year, you will have firmed up relationships with those in your direct team and those you most frequently refer or signpost

DOI: 10.4324/9781003542049-12

too; however, as you settle and embed further within your own practice, you may find benefits in making further links with your wider practitioner family in your locality. Examples of these connections could be:

- EMHPs in other Mental Health Support Teams, to consider any potential sharing of good practice
- PWPs with EMHPs and/or CWPs where they have an adult client with a child needing support, and they are considering signposting advice
- Mental Health Wellbeing Practitioners (MHWPs) with the other practitioner roles to connect with a shared voice when considering role developments

Each region in England, seven in total, has a PPN. These PPNs aim to:

- Engage and connect all psychological professionals in order to support them to have a stronger voice together
- Have an advisory role to policy-makers, workforce planners, and commissioners
- Support the safe and effective expansion of the existing and new psychological professions

PPN membership is open to trainee and qualified psychological professionals, commissioners, other stakeholders, service users, and members of the public. So, this includes any potential, trainee, or qualified PP. Membership is free and comes with a range of benefits.

There is variation in each region's individual offer; however, these include but are not limited to:

- Newsletters with key national and regional information that has an impact on the psychological professions
- Events
- Communities of practice

Here, Chloe Booth shares her experience of joining a PP Community of Practice (CoP). Chloe described the benefits of being involved in the CoP as giving her the opportunity to 'be a voice for the low-intensity workforce' in her region, as well as increasing her opportunities for networking and meeting other PPs outside of her own CWP speciality. These opportunities have supported her to develop as a practitioner:

> I have learnt from others within the low-intensity workforce through the connections I have made in the Community of Practice.
>
> It can feel isolating at times being the only PP within a team or service and being a part of the Community of Practice allows a space to connect with others and feel a part of something valued. It has allowed me the opportunity to be a part of important conversations that are happening regarding the low-intensity workforce.
>
> It has also allowed me to develop additional skills such as increased confidence in public speaking and having something additional and unique to talk about within job interviews.
>
> Importantly, I have been able to develop strong, valued connections with individuals within the low-intensity workforce.
>
> Chloe Booth, Qualified CWP

There are also a variety of other places where practitioners can connect. For example, the British Association of Behavioural and Cognitive Psychotherapies (BABCP) has the Low-Intensity Cognitive Behavioural Interventions SIG (LI SIG). Their aim is to promote and develop low-intensity evidence-based practice and research, whilst supporting the development and opportunities for low-intensity CPD and space for networking and connection. As part of this, the BABCP LI SIG hosts meetings and journal clubs, which are open to BABCP Members.

> I wanted to get involved, in the BABCP LI SIG, because I felt like there was so little out there for Wellbeing Practitioners, that we always felt like an afterthought. I hope the SIG makes a difference by giving a space purely for psychological practitioners, reflecting on the unique challenges these roles bring. We hope to lift the voices of those of us in the profession, so we can shape our development in a way that is led by and suits us.
>
> Sam Torney, Chair BABCP LI SIG

There are also other networking opportunities provided by some of the main CPD providers and other private organisations. When looking for opportunities, we would always just advise practitioners utilise due diligence.

Champion Roles

In our practitioner context, a champion role is broadly defined as a role undertaken by an individual to actively promote and support a specific group or project. The person acts as a point of contact; they may have some additional knowledge, skills, or training but may just have a particular passion or desire to advocate for the area of interest, in order to support it to have the necessary attention and resources drawn to it.

As well as a productive way to channel a particular passion or interest, champion roles can be a great way to add variety into a job plan or begin to develop and build on an area of special interest.

In the National Health Service (NHS) England Talking Therapies (TT) Manual (NHS England, 2024), they reiterate these champion roles as an opportunity to engage in training and CPD, with the opportunity for services to consider the introduction of a champion for specific protected characteristics, digital or staff wellbeing given as examples.

Some of the examples we have seen develop in adult TT services include those for ethnic minority groups, older people, younger adults, perinatal mental health, armed forces veterans, and people with LTCs.

In Children and Young People services, there has been the development of participation champions, Equality Diversity & Inclusion (EDI) champions, and Routine Outcome Measure (ROM) champion type roles.

There is evidence to support that practitioners from across health care who specialise tend to get better results and, in many cases, may have better job satisfaction. So, becoming a champion as you gain experience and confidence in your role is certainly something to consider.

CPD and Further Training

As highlighted in Chapter 11, CPD is a requirement for the registered qualified practitioner in order to maintain their skills and competence but also to develop in their role. To further support development, there are also additional opportunities to engage in official further training that is practitioner-specific.

CPD

The CPD requirements for ongoing registration are available on the BPS and BABCP websites and summarised in Chapter 11 of this book.

Many services will have specific processes for approving CPD; some may even provide or buy in CPD for practitioners; however, you may find yourself in a position where you need to source your own CPD or have a specific personal development need that you identify some CPD for.

When seeking out CPD, you should ensure that it meets your specific needs: Has it been developed for a low-intensity practitioner role? Is it appropriate and suitable for your scope of practice? Has it been developed by a reputable and appropriately qualified person or company?

If it is, enjoy learning, and remember to complete reflective logs for your ongoing registration.

Official Training Courses

Once you have achieved your initial practitioner qualification, there are various options of additional qualifications you can apply to complete.

For PWPs, this includes the NHS TT Supervisor Course. Services commissioned to provide TT can access places on this course for their PWPs through the NHS England Education Training Activity Plan (ETAP) process in conjunction with their Integrated Care Board. This course supports the development of Caseload Management Supervision (CMS) and Clinical Skills Supervision (CSS) competencies. PWPs should have at least one year of qualified clinical experience and undertake and pass this course in order to be able to deliver CMS and CSS. This is often a requirement as a Senior PWP (SPWP); however, experienced PWPs can also complete this course and provide CMS/CSS.

The course explores the role of supervision for both the organisation and the profession, as well as the development of reflective practice. Skills in the competencies to deliver effective CMS and CSS including the ability to identify and manage concerns, the impact of relationships, and supervision of intervention are also covered. The course is most commonly delivered as five days, and as part of the assessment, the SPWP/PWP is required to submit a recording of themselves delivering CMS/CSS.

PWP can also access the LTC top-up training. The NHS TT manual (NHS England, 2024) recommends that PWPs complete the LTC top-up training, for PWPs, within two years of completing the initial PWP course. The LTC training provides knowledge on specified conditions as well as supporting the development of skills to work with those clients with LTCs. The conditions identified in the curriculum (NHS England, 2023) to be covered in the training are long-term physical conditions such as diabetes, cardiac disease, respiratory disease, cancer with accompanying low mood and/or anxiety, neurological conditions (sudden onset, e.g., stroke, intermittent conditions, e.g., epilepsy, progressive conditions, e.g., Parkinson's, and stable conditions with changing needs, e.g., cerebral palsy), and long-COVID. Like the TT Supervisor Course, services commissioned to provide TT can access places on this course for their PWPs through the METP process.

More recently, there has also been the development offers such as the PGDip/GradDip Enhanced Psychological Therapies Practice (low-intensity cognitive behavioural therapy (CBT)) for PWPs; these courses are being designed to support the growth and development of PWPs looking to further their careers within the roles, that is, SPWPs and Service Leads. These courses are not currently on the ETAP and are subject to PWPs being able to secure funding and support from their employing organisation. As well as covering aspects related to supervision, this course covers topics designed to extend, enhance, and adapt evidence-based practice and develop leadership and service development skills.

For CWPs and EMHPs, there has been the development of the SWP postgraduate diploma. The course design supports CWPs and EMHPs together with a focus on a shift towards a more individual formulation-based approach, rather than a purely manualised one, to drive treatment. Becoming a SWP is much more about completing a fuller assessment, formulating, and then considering what can be done within the practitioners' low-intensity framework and skill set, and how to adapt the interventions for individual young people; however, it is also about being able to judge where the presentation is not within the SWP competencies for treatment.

> I think there are a range of things that this course introduces that gives [CWPs/EMHPs] a broader spectrum of different interventions and skills. Particularly encouraging thinking about adapting practise and making environmental adjustments. And just knowing more about neurodiversity and learning disability in children and young people.
>
> Charlotte Temple, CWP, EMHP, SWP, Supervisor and
> HI CBT Specialist Lecturer, Clinical Supervisor,
> and CBT therapist

Charlotte has supported the overview of this course curriculum; however, the reader should be aware that the delivery may vary slightly between the higher education institutions commissioned to deliver this course.

Most frequently comprising four modules, the course is taught over one or two years. This can be done one module at a time or through an integrated timetable where multiple modules are taught simultaneously.

Modules 1 and 2 focus on the development of supervision skills, similar to the (TT) Supervisor Course for PWPs, allowing the SWP to take on that specific aspect of supervising.

Module 3 is focused on upskilling through enhanced practice and could be seen as adding to the CWP and EMHPs toolkit, for example, interventions for obsessive compulsive disorder.

The course also considers trauma; Charlotte is very clear that the CWPs and EMHPs are not being taught to deliver trauma-focused CBT or eye movement desensitisation and reprocessing therapy, as a high-intensity CBT therapist would. Rather, SWPs are developing skills to be able to adapt, practice, and work with a trauma-informed approach.

Module 4 is all about adapting their practise for neurodiversity and learning disabilities. The latest research is showing that approximately 90% of Emotionally Based School Avoidance cases in schools are with young people who are neurodiverse, so this is a really important topic. Module 4 teaching has a focus around making reasonable adjustments, thinking about the environment, that is, in their education setting, and understanding the types and needs of neurodiverse conditions and learning disabilities. There are also some overlaps here with the trauma-informed care work.

At the time of writing, there are currently no specific MHWP post-qualification courses, due to the much more recent development of this role; however, this is a fast-paced area of development, and despite the core differences between the roles, there is much shared learning to be gained going forward to the development of career pathways and learning for MHWPs.

Becoming a Senior

Becoming a 'Senior' could be considered a natural progression in the career of a practitioner. It presents a lovely opportunity to not only develop personally from a professional point of view (as well as the financial uplift – SPWP/SWPs are paid at Agenda for Change Band 6), but to support your newer practitioner colleagues and trainees, which can be very rewarding. However, it could also be seen as a challenge to with the responsibilities of the role, such as supervising, enhanced practice, and potential involvement in leadership initiatives and service developments. It is therefore recommended that a practitioner should ideally gain two years of experience post-qualification, in order to consolidate their skills and competencies.

However, as referenced above in 'Official Training Courses', there are some variations in the route to becoming a senior practitioner between the roles. For EMHPs and CWPs, there is the expectation to acquire the Senior Wellbeing Practitioner qualification or supervisor training, whereas, for PWPs, there is the requirement for those with an interest in progressing to a senior post to access the training available for developing supervisory skills (CLM and CSS).

Below are some examples and experiences of those who are or have moved to senior roles to help you further develop a sense of the roles and how they can be challenging but rewarding careers and, in some cases like Adam below, can change your perspective as a practitioner:

I am back at university training to become a senior EMHP and therefore am now a trainee supervisor. This has profoundly transformed my view of supervision, meaning it feels even more valuable now and I recognise just how essential it is, especially as the supervisor of a trainee.

Adam Hope, Qualified EMHP

Sian has been a SPWP for just over three years but has been a PWP for 17 years:

Being a Senior PWP is something I aspired to be for a number of years. I have been in the post a few years now, I feel that it is a good role for both clinical and some operational matters without being a part of the wider management structure.

I enjoy being able to impart my knowledge of the PWP role to others, offer supervision, problem solve situations, create a good team dynamic and be the voice of the PWPs themselves within the wider leadership team.

I love learning from the newer PWP's as it has been some-time since I qualified and love learning a different perspective of the Low Intensity Interventions and approaches.

We get to maintain a clinical approach as well with carry-ing a small caseload, which is very important as this is the main reason the majority of us came into the role. I enjoy seeing cli-ents recover, learn strategies, see them flourish and give them-selves a new lease of life. I gain that feeling of pride vicariously through supervision and seeing the PWPs get the praise that they really deserve.

It feels like you have a foot in each area – clinical and operational without the responsibility for a large team.

Sian Clements, Senior PWP

Samantha talks about why she chose to progress to the SWP course and what she is enjoying about it:

I feel really fascinated by a lot of things, and that's what I'm finding on the SWP course, that I absolutely love my university days, it's so interesting! I suppose I've always wanted to learn a bit more… I've always kind of wondered about high intensity CBT and do I want to go into that? I feel like the SWP course is a really nice dip into the water, to see how I feel and how I get on with the enhanced practice elements.

But there's also the supervision element to it, and I've just had some really amazing supervisors and have wanted to, hopefully, be that for someone else.

Samantha Taylor, trainee SWP (CWP)

Managing Personal Wellbeing

I think the majority of us go into this profession because we care. Sometimes we can care too much, and this can lead to burn out if not properly managed.

Kelly DeSantis, LTC-trained PWP

Many people may pick up this book having read or heard a variety of comments about the roles and their impact on personal wellbeing, similar to Kelly's above, or may go on to do so as they further research the roles. As authors, Kirsty and Elspeth are keen to acknowledge and not shy away from the fact that these roles and their training are demanding. The term 'high volume, low intensity' was coined for the roles and implies a lot.

In her book, Elizabeth Ruth devotes a chapter to 'PP Wellbeing' discussing the factors that can contribute to potential burnout and compassion fatigue (Ruth & Spiers, 2023). These include, but aren't limited to, targets, complexity, and value.

From anecdotal evidence of working in and liaising with many services, and changes such as the introduction of the two-year funding rule (see Chapter 13), we can see that burnout is a significant contributory cause to practitioners not staying in practitioner roles long, looking to progress to other roles, or to them leaving the profession entirely. The PPN PWP Retention Report (Kell & Baguley 2018) was commissioned due to the 25% turnover rate identified in the 2015/2016 Adult Improving Access to Psychological Therapies Workforce Census Report. It identified three themes:

1 Issues in relation to the PWP roles; salary, registration, workforce diversity, caseload, autonomy and flexibility, fidelity to the model, CPD, and job security
2 PWP Career Progression
3 Issues in relation to team/services including wellbeing, systems, IT, processes, supervision and admin, respect and value of the role, and working relationships with other professionals

The report made nine key recommendations; however, due to a range of factors, probably including a global pandemic, changes in NHS England and changes in provider financial positions and targets, not all of these have been actioned. We can see in the most recent Psychological Professions Workforce Census data (NHS England, 2025) that there is still much to be done with the PP turnover rate at 19.2%, which is 3.8% higher than the psychological professions average.

As much as, it needs acknowledgement, consideration, and support to change unhelpful practices in the system, these 'high-volume, low-intensity' roles can be the 'right intensity' for many clients and, as demonstrated by Sian above, sustainable and long lasting careers for practitioners; however, in order for any career to be sustainable and continue to be rewarding, particularly in the world of healthcare and psychology, you need to ensure that you do what you can too. Considering how you take care of and support yourself is part of this, and that is our focus in this section.

Firstly, it is important to consider the factors within the workplace. Some of these may seem obvious, but we should always ensure that we are meeting these basics, as discussed in other chapter's their importance is recognised with many forming registration requirements.

Book in, prepare for, and actively engage in CLM, CSS, and reflective practice. Your supervisors are there to support and guide you, but you get the most from this when you are open, honest, and prepared. Develop a relationship with your Line Manager too, do they know your aspirations, what you may need support with? If you develop relationships with your managers and supervisors, it is easier to seek support if something unexpected occurs.

There are also other less formal ways of managing your wellbeing in work, for example, 'corridor supervision' – those supportive conversations with your colleagues about tricky cases, taking lunch, and perhaps taking a walk.

As practitioners, we all have a good understanding of Behavioural Activation and the role of behaviour in supporting mood (see the role-specific Chapters 2–5) and the need to not neglect specific groups of activities that may contribute to our sense of pleasure and achievement. These may be found in aspects of our

Table 12.1 Suggestions of wellbeing activities by the authors

Elspeth	Kirsty
Walks – long ones with my friend or in the 'Fairy Glen' with children and the dog	Reading – getting stuck into a good book
Hyrox Training Classes (though not actually to compete!)	Creating things… … baking, sewing, crochet, etc.
Planned evenings out with friends – making sure we find time (despite conflicting and hectic schedules) to catch up	Weekends away, either city breaks or campervan trips, or visiting friends

work; however, it is important in the busy role of the practitioner to have focus (pleasure and achievements) outside of work.

As we are all individuals, it is impossible to provide a definitive list of 'wellbeing' activities that will suit everyone; it is important to reflect on what you find beneficial and then consider how you incorporate it into your lifestyle. For a little inspiration, but not as the right or only answers Elspeth and Kirsty share their top threes in Table 12.1:

We would always encourage proactive management of wellbeing, but acknowledge this is not always possible, and there may be some circumstances that require additional or immediate support. All NHS Trusts will provide access to wellbeing services, usually accessed through line management and HR, although many organisations will have self-referral routes to at least some of their options. Other employer organisations offers and referral pathways may vary, but, in all cases, personal GPs will be able to advise and/or signpost to local options of advice and support.

Box 12.1 References and wider reading

BABCP Wellbeing Practitioner Registration. https://babcp.com/Wellbeing-Registrations/About

BPS Wider Psychological Workforce Register. https://www.bps.org.uk/wider-psychological-workforce

Kell, L., & Baguley, C. (2018). *What factors impact on the retention of psychological wellbeing practitioners?:*

Report of a survey into second destination & retention of PWPs. Psychological Professions Network.

NHS England. (2023). *NHS talking therapies: National curriculum for psychological wellbeing practitioners to deliver low intensity interventions in the context of long term persistent and distressing health conditions.* NHS England.

NHS England. (2024). *NHS talking therapies for anxiety and depression manual. 7th Edition.* NHS England. https:// www.england.nhs.uk/wp-content/uploads/2018/06/nhs-talking-therapies-manual-v7.1-updated.pdf

NHS England. (2025). *Psychological professions national workforce census.* NHS England. https://www.england.nhs. uk/publication/psychological-professions-workforce-census/

Psychological Professions Network (PPN). https://ppn. nhs.uk/about-us/who-we-are

Ruth, E., & Spiers, J. (2023). *A pragmatic guide to low intensity psychological therapy: Care in high volume.* Academic Press.

Chapter 13

Thinking about Next Steps

Introduction

Our key message for the start of this chapter will be 'you don't need to leave'. As already referenced in Chapter 12, psychological practitioner (PP) roles can be rewarding careers in their own right! Remaining as a PP, perfecting your skills and delivering psychologically informed care to your clients at their point of need, is an immensely rewarding role.

However, after a period of time, you may wish to think about and explore potential next steps, especially in light of the growing number of career development opportunities that have become available as the PP roles embed and develop within the system.

This chapter will explore the roles that allow individuals to stay within the profession in the broad sense, but allow for the expansion of an individual's own personal journey within the wider offer of opportunities available and their ability to have a variety of different impacts through these, whilst still being able to utilise skills they developed as a PP.

These other opportunities currently vary between PP professions and geographical locations, though there does appear to be momentum and appetite for these opportunities and developments across all the roles and regions. To introduce these, and in acknowledgement of the current differing positions between PP roles, we have grouped them into themes of development opportunities – leadership, education, research, and writing.

In relation to clinical opportunities, we are aware of acknowledging those who may wish to explore additional clinical training; therefore, looking beyond their PP role, for example, to the clinical

DOI: 10.4324/9781003542049-13

psychology doctorate or to becoming a cognitive behavioural therapist or high-intensity therapist (HIT). In acknowledging this, it is crucial that we highlight the National Health Service England (NHSE) two-year funding rule, and we will discuss this below. The more specific details of these alternative clinical routes will be discussed in Chapter 14. This will allow us to place them in context, as they are not PP roles, which is the main focus of this text.

Policy Context

When Improving Access to Psychological Therapies (IAPT) was first introduced and rolled out across England, there was little consideration of career progression for the newly established PP role (Psychological Wellbeing Practitioners (PWPs)). They trained at Agenda for Change (AfC) Band 4 and moved to AfC Band 5 as Qualified PWPs, but there was a ceiling. To further progress clinically or financially required PWPs to leave their substantive positions and seek alternative career routes. This position was potentially amplified by the lack of understanding of the role, competencies, and potential of this new workforce.

Over the past 16 years, this narrative has shifted, our PP workforce has much to offer, and this has been recognised in IAPT, now known as NHS Talking Therapies for anxiety and depression (NHS TTad). In NHS TTad, there has been the development of a number of clinical roles, such as Senior PWPs (SPWPs), specialist PWPs, deputy, and clinical lead roles, in addition to job descriptions and personal specifications going through AfC matching to allow applications from PWPs into operational roles such as team leads and service managers.

These developments have also been picked up over shorter time frames in other PP roles, for example, Children's Wellbeing Practitioners (CWPs) and Education Mental Health Practitioners (EMHPs) being able to train to become Senior Wellbeing Practitioners (SWPs); see Chapter 12 for further details about this course. However, there is still significant variation within and between roles and regions, with the pace of change varying, partly in relation to the time since the inception of the individual roles, but also impacted by system issues, such as team skill mix and needs, that is, for SWPs.

From a policy and service perspective, this reflection on developments is also relevant in relation to the NHS Long-Term Workforce Plan (LTWP) aims around retention. The NHS LTWP, published in June 2023, is the most comprehensive NHS workforce document ever produced. It provides details on the expectations for training, retaining, and reforming the NHS workforce in England. This includes the necessary requirements for growth of the NHS Workforce between 2021/2022 and 2036/2037. The King's Fund has some articles which explore this expansion and its implications in more detail (Holden, 2023). Within this expansion, the psychological professions account for the biggest and fastest growth (Psychological Professions Benchmarking Data). To support this growth, we need to retain our qualified PPs, valuing their work, allowing them to become experienced colleagues, and, where appropriate, supporting them to develop, to be able to support, nurture, supervise, and lead the cohorts of trainees that need to follow.

There are already some fantastic examples of PPs who have carved out varied career journeys based on their initial PP skills and competencies, for example, Jordan below:

Being a PWP has been fundamental in my journey to becoming a HIT and Supervision Lead. It was challenging at times, but the skills, experience and knowledge I gained were invaluable to me. In my current role, I am privileged to be able support other therapists in developing their own clinical skills and confidence. I feel the PWP role has been integral for me in being able to do this to the best of my ability.

Jordan Howarth, Qualified PWP and
HIT. Now a Supervision Lead in a
large Talking Therapies Service

Leadership

What is leadership? What makes a good leader? Is a manager the same as a leader or different, encompassing of leadership qualities or with a distinct skill set? There are many books devoted entirely to this subject, and we will not be able to answer them here. But these are important questions to reflect on, if you feel this may be a career route you wish to explore.

Many organisations have a hierarchical approach to management and leadership structures. The impact of factors such as AfC and 'Core Professions' in the NHS has historically meant that these managerial and leadership roles have been dominated by particular professions, such as doctors, nurses, and clinical psychologists. However, as mentioned, we are seeing a shift, with more reflection being taken on role competencies and skills mix of teams, rather than traditional titles, further influenced by vacancy rates and recruitment issues in some professions. These shifts are beginning to be reflected in personal specifications and job descriptions for leadership and managerial roles.

Through conversations with Sam Torney (who we've met in Chapter 7, a team lead and PWP by background) and her team of PWPs, it was clear to see how 'having leadership who have practitioner background can be exceptionally supportive' works in practice and to see the value of PPs finding their place in the world of leadership and management.

Robyn Ward is a qualified CWP, low-intensity supervisor, and trainee HI CBT therapist. Robyn tells us she completed an introduction to supervision course initially, before going on to the PG Cert programme in LI supervision. Robyn shares, "I got a lot out of that course because it pushed me outside of my comfort zone. I had to learn about models of supervision, and think about how to supportively challenge".

Robyn also tells us that, through working in a senior role in her team, she has been able to develop some leadership skills, saying

It's given me a bit more drive to think about how we can better ourselves as a team and how we can use data to support this, know what we need to work towards, and think about how we can meet the needs of our community as a LI service.

Broadly speaking, in the NHS, we can divide these roles between operational management and clinical leadership. We know that PPs, from their training and clinical experience (also see Chapter 7), have a range of transferable skills that can aid them in these roles.

Operational Management

Examples of operational management roles in the NHS teams that PPs may have contact with or aspire to can include job titles such as team lead and service manager, though there may be variations or additional titles within the NHS or in the non-NHS organisations that employ PPs.

These management roles will often comprise responsibilities and tasks related to the interpretation of data, the achievement of targets, and the management of finances and staffing. The workforce elements within this are likely to include tasks, such as line management, recruitment, and absence management.

> After 12 months of working as a qualified PWP I applied for the Senior PWP role. I found that I enjoyed stepping away from clinical work with patients and focussing on supporting staff more than I thought I would. Working in the Senior role and developing more supervisory/management skills made me want to progress in a more managerial role rather than going down the HIT route.
>
> I applied for a team lead role and at the time there were a lot of changes in the service and to the role that I initially applied for. It was a challenging 2 years, but I have really enjoyed working with staff and supporting them to be able to come to work and carry out their roles to the best of their abilities.
>
> I feel like my previous work as a PWP and Senior PWP was a really good foundation to becoming a team lead, I had previous knowledge of Step 2 work plans, diaries, training needs and supervision. I was able to transfer this knowledge over to Step 3 when managing Step 3 staff as well.
>
> For me the part of the job that I enjoy the most is line management and supporting staff. Again, I feel that my previous work as a PWP has helped me with this in terms of being able to problem solve, try to prevent burnout and looking after the physical/mental health of staff whilst carrying out a really busy role.
>
> Stacy Smith, Team Lead and Qualified PWP

As referenced, there is some variation in the levels of development for CWPs and EMHPs into operational roles; however, Lettie Smyth, a qualified and experienced CWP and qualified low-intensity supervisor, holds some line management responsibility within their team, showing that there is potential for this career pathway for PPs. Lettie tells us, "I think it's been good for our team because it gives senior members of staff more variety of responsibility. It also opens up opportunities for those who might want to develop strategically".

Clinical

Clinical leadership holds different responsibilities to operational leadership, with the focus on, but not limited to, clinical decision-making, governance, and supervision. The types of clinical leadership roles may include senior PPs (covered in Chapter 12), specialist PPs, for example, long-term conditions focussed, and deputy clinical lead, and clinical leads. The level of clinical leadership also influences the specific tasks and responsibilities. Seniors, for example, may focus on the day to day, including tasks such as clinical management supervision, with a clinical lead more focussed on the professional leadership and strategic direction of the service. There is much anecdotal evidence of the benefits of having experienced PPs in these roles, with PPs feeling heard, valued, and supported.

> Having the opportunity to progress into a PWP Clinical Lead role has been a privilege and something that I am extremely grateful for. I couldn't have progressed into the role without the support of the organisation that I work for, who have helped me develop from a PWP following qualification in 2015, to becoming a Senior PWP in 2017, to then being offered my current post in 2019. Being a PWP Clinical Lead is so rewarding and I enjoy the variety that the role offers, meaning that I can still work clinically with patients, whilst also supporting other PWPs within their roles with their own development and overseeing our Step 2 pathway.
>
> Sarah Barker, PWP Clinical Lead (Step 2 Pathway),
> qualified PWP and LTC trained

Educator Roles

Although a more experienced PP may take on an informal education role (perhaps of trainees) or an in-service delivery of continuing professional development session role (i.e., for more junior PPs), here we are considering the progression to more formal teaching in academia.

Initially, this may be as a lecturer or a tutor, delivering course content, assessing practice, and so on, with some of these roles being offered part-time alongside ongoing contracts as practicing PPs.

> Having been employed as a PWP within the NHS and moving into a Senior PWP role for several years, I started to identify that my skills and interests were in line with supporting trainees and qualified staff to learn and develop. I am passionate about the role of a PWP and wanted to share my knowledge and skills with those who were on this career path. I have now been teaching at a university on the PGCert Primary Care Mental Health for 4 years and feel that the skills I developed as a qualified PWP have supported the transition into this role.
>
> These skills include things such as development for wellbeing groups within step 2, ensuring that the content is informed by the evidence and literature for step 2 interventions. Delivering didactic groups as a PWP developed my skills at presenting to larger audiences and how to maintain engagement which has helped with lecture delivery. Supervising both qualified and trainee PWPs enabled me to stay relevant and ensure my practice is in line with NICE guidance which is transferrable to building content for my lectures at the university. Within supervision, role play would be observed and feedback given to PWPs which is transferrable to skills practice at the university where I provide structured feedback to students on their practice.
>
> My experiences of working with a diverse range of patients in practice, and engagement of a perinatal champion role within service has supported me in my transition to Unit lead of the values, diversity, and context unit on the university programme. This has allowed me to bring authenticity of someone who has worked clinically in services as a qualified PWP, this has been invaluable for trainee development at the university. Working in higher education teaching students to become PWP's has felt like a natural career progression for me and

allowed me to continue my career within psychological well-being which is where my passion remains.

Bryony Beetham, Lecturer, NHS TT Team Lead,
and Qualified PWP

There are also examples of progression of PPs within academic roles, such as to programme lead roles.

Research and Writing

Our PP roles were designed to deliver evidence-based practice. To continue to develop the field further, we need to continue to build our evidence base. This is done through research.

This may predominantly be university-based studies, but here we could also consider the opportunities on going in services, such as quality improvement projects, which could potentially be written up and the good practice or learning shared.

There are multiple outlets that may allow opportunity to share written pieces, for example, newsletters and blogs to formal submission of written articles to journals or governing body magazines.

For more formal journal publications, there are specific guidelines to adhere too, and articles will go through a peer-review process. Here, Eve, a qualified PWP by background, describes her experience of being a peer reviewer:

One of my areas of interest is low-intensity representation in research, and I am a peer reviewer for The Cognitive Behaviour Therapist. Peer reviewing is a fantastic way to develop your academic and research-related skills as a low-intensity PP, and to expand and deepen your own practice too. Peer reviewing supports the publishing of the best quality research. When a piece of work gets submitted to the journal, the handling editor invites selected reviewers to contribute, based on your experience and expertise, so I provide input from a low-intensity perspective but can also contribute to papers more broadly about CBT. The process of peer reviewing requires a lot of considerations. When I review a piece of work I am thinking about whether it makes a contribution to the low-intensity profession and how well the authors explain it. I also think about whether the data and arguments presented are sound and accurate, and if the piece of work has clear aims and conclusions that will help develop low-intensity practice. This sometimes means I have to go off and read other papers to make sure I understand references being used or think about how the piece of work would apply in my own practice. Not all journals are just original research, so things like clinical guidance papers are a great way to support acquiring knowledge and procedural skills too. I always come away from the process feeling very inspired, wanting to do more reading, and thinking about how I can improve my own practice!

> Eve Bampton-Wilton, Senior Lecturer and Clinical
> Programme Manager in the Psychological
> Professions Network (PPN) South West
> and qualified PWP

There are also opportunities to write in other published formats; contribute quotes, chapters, or even write whole books (like this one!)

Moving to Other Clinical Roles

The remit of this book is focussed on the PP roles; however, the authors are aware that, for some, the natural progression will be to explore a transition to another clinical role. Or having read this book, you may be considering whether there is another role that would better suit your clinical interests or skill set.

For these reasons, Chapter 14 will outline and briefly consider some of the other related clinical roles, in order to support PPs, or PPs to be, in making an informed choice about their career path.

For those in other professional or operational roles reading this book to increase their broader understanding of the PP roles, it is important to and will be helpful in supporting understanding around 'which role do I need' considering clinical competencies of each role and how these may interface, overlap, or differ.

For those for whom progression to another clinical role is the route that you are considering, there are two key issues outlined here that require understanding.

NHS England Two-Year Funding Rule

The two-year funding rule was introduced in April 2022 (Health Education England, 2022). This policy change impacts on individuals looking to undertake more than one NHS-funded psychological professions training programme. Individuals who have completed an NHS-funded psychological professions training programme will not be eligible to complete a further funded training programme until a minimum of two years after the qualifying exam board of the previous training programme. The rule applies to anyone who starts a course, whether they complete or not.

Knowledge, Skills, and Attitudes (KSA) Document

Some of the clinical career progression roles would, depending on prior qualifications, require a PP to complete a KSA document. Those who do not have a recognised core profession (i.e., mental health nurse or social worker) are required to complete the KSA in order to demonstrate the ability to embark on high-intensity training. There is a shortened version for those who have completed a psychology degree eligible for British Psychological Society (BPS) Graduate Basis for Registration and have been registered

Table 13.1 Summary of KSA portfolio areas

Knowledge	Skills	Attitudes
Life stages and human development	Competency in key relationship skills	Fitness to practice and suitable at a personal level
Health and social care approaches	Maintain and manage records and reports	Self-evaluation and reflection
Psychopathology/ diagnostic skills	Communication with services and colleagues	Has an enquiring mind and is receptive to the scientist PP approach
Models of therapy	Awareness of risk	Biography or clinical experience record
	Comprehension of research	
	Commitment to ethical principles	

as a PP on the BPS or British Association of Behavioural and Cognitive Psychotherapists Wellbeing Practitioner registers.

The document comprises building a portfolio of evidence, or training and experience, which allows the individual completing it to demonstrate equivalence to having a core profession. This experience should have been achieved over at least a four-year period.

The portfolio covers the areas shown in Table 13.1.

Evidence for each of the areas should come from a range of sources including training, references, and self-directed study.

Box 13.1 References and wider reading

British Association of Behavioural and Cognitive Psychotherapies. *Knowledge, skills and attitudes.* https://babcp.com/core-professions/knowledge-skills-attitudes/

Health Education England. (2022). *NHS funding for psychological professions training programmes.* HEE. https://www.hee.nhs.uk/our-work/mental-health/psychological-professions/nhs-funding-psychological-professions-training-programmes

Holden, J. (2023). *The NHS long term workforce plan explained.* The King's Fund. https://www.kingsfund.org.uk/insight-and-analysis/long-reads/nhs-long-term-workforce-plan-explained

NHS England. (2023). *NHS long term workforce plan.* NHS England.

Chapter 14

Related Roles

Introduction

The practitioner landscape has seen significant development over the last 15 years, and the landscape continues to evolve. This chapter explores this wider landscape, as we know, when it comes to your career, you want to make an informed choice and understand all the options available to you.

Whilst we hope you have been inspired by the psychological practitioner (PP) careers we have outlined in this book, there are also ALL the other psychological professional roles; those reading this book at the beginning their journey within the field of psychology may wish to consider further research of these alternatives, particularly if they have or are considering studying for an undergraduate psychology degree; therefore, we are including a brief overview of some of these here, particularly ones also considered by some to be practitioner career progression options.

Psychological Professions Taxonomy

The psychological professions is a large group, with far more individual professions than most people realise. The psychological professions taxonomy, at the time of publication, lists 19 distinct psychological professions roles.

These are split into three main categories:

- Psychological practitioners
- Psychological therapists
- Psychologists

DOI: 10.4324/9781003542049-14

Within these categories, there are then a number of roles, see Table 14.1.

Within a category, there are similarities between the roles; however, each of these roles has its own training and competencies.

We would encourage any aspiring psychological professional to consider the importance of their own individual skills,

Table 14.1 Taxonomy of the Psychological Professions

Taxonomy of Psychological Professions

Psychological Practitioners	Psychological Therapists	Psychologists	Associate and Assistant Roles
Psychological Wellbeing Practitioner	Cognitive Behavioural Therapists	Clinical Psychologists	Clinical Associate in Psychology
Education Mental Health Practitioner	Counsellors	Counselling Psychologists	Assistant Psychologist
Children's Wellbeing Practitioner	Child and Adolescent Psychotherapists	Forensic Psychologists	
Mental Health and Wellbeing Practitioner	Adult Psychotherapists	Health Psychologists	
Youth Intensive Psychological Practitioner (pilot programme)	Family and Systemic Psychotherapists		
	Psychological Therapists (Other)		
	Art, Drama, and Music Therapists (with AHP Professional Leadership)		
	Medical Psychotherapists (with Medical Professional Leadership)		

experience, and aspirations – Chapter 7 may also help you to think about and reflect on this. You should then consider how you wish to apply these skills and experiences, in order to support informed choice, within your aspirational ideas, and hopefully allow you to progress in a role that suits you best as an individual and that you will find rewarding.

In addition to this book's information, the Psychological Professions Network (PPN) has developed a Careers Map, which is a really great resource for aspiring psychological professionals to support informed decision-making. The PPN Careers Map gives information about roles in the taxonomy. You can browse the whole map or search for more tailored roles by selecting the type of qualification you already have.

The National Health Service (NHS) Health Careers website is another trustworthy source of information. This resource has a much broader remit, allowing people to access information not only on the psychological professions but all 350+ NHS Careers, including Allied Health Professions (AHPs). This website includes information on the different role remits and entry requirements for the many and varied health profession careers. If 350+ careers feels overwhelming, there is a 'find your career' quiz, and once you've located a role you are interested in, there are links to live vacancies, for many roles.

Other Psychological Roles

In this book, we have focused specifically on the PP roles; there are many other books and resources, including ones in this British Psychological Society (BPS) series that focus on other psychological professions. Below, we only provide the briefest of summaries, by way of illustration, of a selection of the most commonly occurring alternatives or clinical progressions for those considering moving on from or as an alternative to a practitioner role.

We would love to have inspired you to pursue or further explore PP roles, but, as referenced in the taxonomy above, there are also other routes that can be taken. What we would encourage, if you do not feel any of the practitioner roles suit you and your skill set, is that you consider one of the many other roles that are available within the psychological professions, not just becoming the 'Clinical Psychologist' most people first think of first.

We met Rob first in Chapter 7, considering the variety of backgrounds practitioners can come from and how this can benefit the workforce and the populations we serve. Rob is an example of a practitioner who has developed their clinical career but sees value still in his initial practitioner training and experience:

> I thoroughly enjoyed my PWP training and went on to be employed as a PWP. I feel the skills I gained as a PWP and counsellor complemented each other and gave me a solid foundation to become a confident therapist. I have now added to this skill set, firstly through training and working as a CBT therapist, and also working my way up to becoming an EMDR Consultant. I am now a Supervision Lead for a Talking Therapies service and have a small private practice of CBT and EMDR patients. I believe my PWP experience has given me the necessary skill set to pursue this career pathway.
>
> Rob Leigh, NHS Talking Therapies (NHSTT) Supervision Lead, a qualified Psychological Wellbeing Practitioner (PWP), High-Intensity Cognitive Behavioural Therapist (HIT CBT), and Eye Movement Desensitisation and Reprocessing (EMDR) Consultant.

Rob's career path demonstrates how a practitioner role can be a really good foundation for some of these other psychological professions.

High-Intensity Therapist (HIT) Roles

HIT was a term coined in Improving Access to Psychological Therapies (IAPT) Services, now known as NHSTT. Initially, most of those HIT roles in IAPT were cognitive behavioural therapy (CBT) therapists. You'll see much more diversity these days in HIT, in NHS TT; there are also CBT roles and other HITs in Children's and Young People's services.

The title 'HIT', in NHS TT, encompasses therapists trained in CBT, Counselling for Depression, Dynamic Interpersonal Therapy, Couples Therapy for Depression, and Interpersonal Therapy. There are also HITs trained in EMDR.

These different modalities all have their own prerequisite training requirements and post-qualification accreditation and continuing professional development requirements.

All these roles would fall under Psychological Therapist in our psychological professions taxonomy.

Workforce data shows that the HIT CBT therapist role is one of the most common and popular career pathway development for many PWPs, developing their career within NHS TT.

Scope

HIT CBT therapists are trained to work with adults (16+ years) within NHS TT Step 3. They work collaboratively with their clients to make changes to improve their mood and mental health. Presentations include anxiety disorders (i.e., social anxiety, post-traumatic stress disorder, obsessive compulsive disorder, and health anxiety) and depression.

HIT CBT therapists utilise hour-long treatment sessions, usually weekly, for an average of 12–20 sessions, but should be led by the National Institute for Health and Care Excellence Guidelines.

Interventions

In Chapter 13, we met Jordan (Supervision Lead in an NHS TT service, a qualified PWP, and a HIT CBT); here, he describes CBT and the role of the HIT CBT therapist:

> CBT helps clients to understand and change unhelpful thoughts, behaviours, and other patterns that may contribute to the maintenance of emotional distress, such as depression and anxiety. It is a practical, goal-focused therapy and is based on a shared understanding of a client's difficulties, which often comes in form of an individualised formulation.
>
> CBT is not a passive therapy, and it encourages active participation and engagement in out of sessions tasks which may include regular behavioural experiments, exposure exercises and utilisation of other taught skills such as cognitive restructuring.

CBT therapists use evidence-based and manualised protocols within their treatments, however therapists will often apply these manuals flexibly whilst being guided by the formulation.

Qualification, Accreditation, and Pay

Access to training requires the individual to have a core profession, or if a PWP with no core profession, a Knowledge, Skills, and Attitudes portfolio can be completed. There is a shortened version for practitioners who have a psychology degree. See Chapter 13 for further information.

Currently, you are able to apply to train on NHS-funded training courses, with places being advertised as trainee HIT CBT roles. If taking this route, individuals complete their university training days alongside placement within NHS TT.

Once qualified, HIT CBTs are required to achieve and maintain accreditation with the British Association of Behavioural and Cognitive Psychotherapies.

The role is paid at an Agenda for Change (AfC) Band 6, whilst in training and upon qualification, individuals are paid at AfC Band 7.

Clinical Associate in Applied Psychology (CAAPs) and Clinical Associate in Psychology (CAPs)

Acronyms in the psychological professions' world, are often confusing, and none more so than the two roles: CAP and CAAP.

As with the other roles within this chapter, we are only giving a brief summary, but I think it's important here to try and differentiate between these two new, interesting and exciting role developments within the psychological professions.

The CAAP role was first developed in Scotland and more recently in Wales. The CAAP role is different from the role of a CAP that has been more recently developed in England. This is because the context in Scotland and Wales is different as those two nations do not have PWP, Mental Health and Wellbeing Practitioner, Children's Wellbeing Practitioner, and Education Mental Health Practitioner roles.

We will first have a quick look at the CAAP role in Scotland and Wales, and then we will go on to look at the CAP role, the role you'll find in England.

CAAP Scope

In Scotland and Wales, the service context is different; you will not find the equivalent of NHS TT, and there are other service differences there as well. The CAAP role was developed to fulfil a gap and requirement for psychologically informed care and provision.

As a CAAP, you train either to work with adults in primary care and adult mental health services or to work with children, young people, and families.

The CAAP role is designed to reduce stress and improve psychological wellbeing, treating conditions such as low mood and mild to moderate anxiety and depression. CAAPs working with children may cover issues such as behavioural and adjustment difficulties.

Interventions

CAAPs are trained to deliver evidence-based support and can use research skills to carry out evaluations.

Qualification and Pay

An undergraduate degree in psychology is a requirement. The CAAP training itself is a one-year MSc in Applied Psychology. As previously stated, this specialises in either primary care and adult mental health or children, young people, and families.

On qualification, CAAPs are paid at AfC Band 7.

CAP Scope

The CAP role is in England. Initially developed in the South West, in 2021, in response to clinical needs and adapted from the implemented CAAP role in Scotland. The CAP role was designed to fulfil a competency gap between Assistant Psychologists and Clinical Psychologists.

Further information on the development of the CAP role, in England, can be found on the Skills for Health website in a presentation by Laidlow (2021).

Interventions

The CAP's core competencies are in the following areas:

- Assessment
- Formulation
- Intervention
- Evaluation
- Research communication
- Professional and values-based practice

The academic curriculum provides CAPs with knowledge in relation to the fundamentals of applied professional psychological practice. As well as their generic competencies, the CAPs develop population-specific competencies based on their work setting placement during training, for example, autism pathway.

Qualification and Pay

CAP training is through the degree apprenticeship route. On qualification, a CAP is qualified to work with a specific client group; this will be where they have completed their clinical work whilst training.

CAPs train at an AfC Band 5 and, upon qualification, are paid at an AfC Band 6.

Clinical Psychologist

A Clinical Psychologist in the taxonomy is in the category of Practitioner Psychologist. When speaking about psychological professions careers to children, young people, and even the general public, often the first and sometimes only role that they come back with is a Clinical Psychologist. We know from what we have already read in this chapter that this is not the case. The taxonomy has 18 other roles, including other Practitioner Psychologists – Health, Counselling, and Forensic. But it would be remiss not to mention here the Doctorate in Clinical Psychology.

It is the longest-standing psychological profession, and as the PP roles have grown and developed, it has also been seen as a career progression move for some. Other routes on to the Doctorate in Clinical Psychology include, but are not limited to, those who have undertaken assistant psychologist or research assistant roles.

Applications for the Doctorate in Clinical Psychology are highly competitive. Applications for the 30 course providers are managed by the Clearing House, with the system opening for new applications each September.

Scope

You will find Clinical Psychologists employed in a whole range of settings and working with a whole range of different populations, from primary care, secondary care, and tertiary care in the NHS to private practice.

Clinical Psychologists train to work with all ages and on a wide range of psychological difficulties, in both mental and physical health. This can include anxiety, depression, psychosis, personality disorder, eating disorders, addictions, learning disabilities, and family or relationship issues.

They can be found working with individuals, as well as teams and organisations to develop and support psychological practice.

Interventions

Clinical Psychologists will use formulation and develop individualised treatment plans for their clients. They will also often undertake additional modality-specific trainings, incorporating these skills into their practice.

They will often also provide consultation on cases and supervision within the teams that they work in.

Clinical Psychologists' job plans usually include more than just direct clinical work; they may be involved in research, audit, and service development and/or hold leadership responsibilities.

Qualification, Accreditation, and Pay

A Clinical Psychologist who is qualified to a doctoral level will have previously completed an undergraduate degree in psychology, accredited by the BPS. Or there is the option of BPS-approved conversion courses, if the first undergraduate degree isn't in psychology or accredited with the BPS. Applicants often have got additional clinical and research experience.

The doctorate is delivered over three years with university teaching, clinical placements, and a thesis.

As previously mentioned, applications for the doctorate course are made through the Clearing House. The course is highly competitive, and the BPS has a publication titled the Alternative Handbook, as well as the information available on the Clearing House website, which details vast amounts of information on the courses and process of application and is a brilliant resource, if you felt that this was the route you wished to explore.

Whilst training, trainee Clinical Psychologists are employed by an NHS trust and paid at AfC Band 6. Upon qualification, Clinical Psychologists are paid at Band 7 and above depending on role, responsibilities, and experience.

Clinical Psychologists are regulated and register with the Health and Care Professions Council. But they may also hold additional accreditations based on trainings undertaken.

Conclusion

We hope that this chapter on other roles has been helpful to you.

In highlighting the full range of psychological professions within the taxonomy, albeit briefly, we hope that this helps to allow you to make informed choices within your early career, following up on some of these options in more detail if they are of interest to you.

Box 14.1 References and Wider Reading

Psychological Professions Network Career Map (https://ppn.nhs.uk/resources-url/careers-map)

Psychological Professions Network Psychological Professions Taxonomy (https://www.ppn.nhs.uk/london/about-us/who-are-the-psychological-professions)

NHS Health Careers website (https://www.healthcareers.nhs.uk/explore-roles)

YIPP: Delivering inpatient children and young people's mental health care (https://www.ucl.ac.uk/pals/research/clinical-educational-and-health-psychology/research-groups/core/competence-frameworks-19)

CAP/CAAP Essay (NHS Scotland, 2024)

CAP role, in England, can be found Skills for Health website here in a presentation by Laidlow (2021) the implemented CAAP role (BPS, 2024) in Scotland.

Welcome to the Clearing House for Postgraduate Courses in Clinical Psychology | Clearing house (https://www.clearing-house.org.uk/)

BPS has a publication titled the Alternative Handbook (https://explore.bps.org.uk/content/report-guideline/bpsrep.2023.inf121)

Final Remarks

We hope that you have found this book a useful and informative resource.

In highlighting the range of psychological practitioner roles, including Psychological Wellbeing Practitioner, Mental Health Wellbeing Practitioner, Children's Wellbeing Practitioner, and Education Mental Health Practitioner, our aim was for this to help you make informed choices within your early career.

In relation to psychological professions, we hope that it has inspired you to continue your journey in the psychological professions field – from our point of view, ideally as a psychological practitioner!

As we have said in various chapters throughout this book, think about your own skills:

What makes you unique?

What do you enjoy?

What do you like to be involved in?

Where do you think you may want to contribute?

Use that as the basis for your decision and for your applications. We spend so much of our lives working it's important that we enjoy it. All of the careers that we've mentioned can be highly rewarding, either in their own right or as part of a wider career journey.

We hope that this book has enabled you to start your own journey and wish you all the best with your future career.

Elspeth and Kirsty

DOI: 10.4324/9781003542049-15

Index

For Product Safety Concerns and Information please contact our EU
representative GPSR@taylorandfrancis.com
Taylor & Francis Verlag GmbH, Kaufingerstraße 24, 80331 München, Germany